Close Relationships

What Couple Therapists Can Learn

Susan S. Hendrick

Texas Tech University

Brooks/Cole Publishing Company

I(T)P™ An International Thomson Publishing Company

Pacific Grove • Albany • Bonn • Boston • Cincinnati • Detroit • London • Madrid • Melbourne
Mexico City • New York • Paris • San Francisco • Singapore • Tokyo • Toronto • Washington

A CLAIREMONT BOOK

Sponsoring Editor: *Claire Verduin*
Marketing Representative: *Rusty Johnson*
Editorial Associate: *Gay C. Bond*
Production Editor: *Nancy L. Shammas*
Production Assistant: *Tessa A. McGlasson*
Manuscript Editor: *Kay Mikel*
Permissions Editor: *Elaine Jones*

Interior Design: *Vernon T. Boes*
Cover Design: *Laurie Albrecht*
Indexer: *James Minkin*
Typesetting: *Huse Publications*
Printing and Binding: *Malloy Lithograph-ing, Inc.*

For more information, contact:

BROOKS/COLE PUBLISHING COMPANY
511 Forest Lodge Road
Pacific Grove, CA 93950
USA

International Thomson Publishing Europe
Berkshire House 168–173
High Holborn
London WC1V 7AA
England

Thomas Nelson Australia
102 Dodds Street
South Melbourne, 3205
Victoria, Australia

Nelson Canada
1120 Birchmount Road
Scarborough, Ontario
Canada M1K 5G4

International Thomson Editores
Campos Eliseos 385, Piso 7
Col. Polanco
11560 México D. F. México

International Thomson Publishing GmbH
Königswinterer Strasse 418
53227 Bonn
Germany

International Thomson Publishing Asia
221 Henderson Road #05–10
Henderson Building
Singapore 0315

International Thomson Publishing Japan
Hirakawacho–cho Kyowa Building, 3F
2–2–1 Hirakawacho–cho
Chiyoda–ku, 102 Tokyo
Japan

Printed in the United States of America.

10   9   8   7   6   5   4   3   2   1

Library of Congress Cataloging-in-Publication Data

Hendrick, Susan, 1944-
    Close relationships : what couple therapists can learn / Susan S.
Hendrick.
        p.   cm.
    Includes bibliographical references (p.   ) and index.
    ISBN 0-534-25434-9
    1. Marriage counseling.   2. Unmarried couples—Counseling of.
I. Title.
HQ10.H44   1994   94-26025
362.82'86—dc20   CIP

CONTENTS

To Clyde

PREFACE

This book introduces therapists and therapists-in-training to the developing literature on close, personal relationships. This literature has burgeoned in the past decade, fueled by research in psychology (social, counseling, clinical, and developmental), sociology, human development and family studies, and communication. This multidisciplinary area, which is concerned with people's intimate relationships with romantic partners, family, and friends, has been the subject of numerous books, journals, conferences, and professional associations. However, the area is confined largely to academic scholars and has not yet been communicated to the larger world of practitioners, a problem this book addresses.

Selective close relationships theory and research has been provided that can be applied by therapists and therapists-in-training who work with couples. Clinical examples from couple counseling are used throughout to illustrate conceptual points, and nearly all chapters conclude with an extended couple counseling case example. In addition to close relationships work, material has also been drawn more generally from psychology, sociology, family studies, and marriage and family therapy as needed.

The current volume contains seven chapters that are loosely ordered to approximate relationship initiation and development, relationship maintenance and progression, and relationship dissolution. Chapter 1 provides an introduction to the field of close relationships and to some of the basic considerations in doing couple counseling, including the therapist's relationship with the clients, the early steps in initiating therapy with couples, and some of the theoretical approaches that apply to couple work. Chapter 2 begins the presentation of close relationships research that has applications to couple counseling. Interpersonal attraction, relationship development, and love are discussed. Chapter 3 is concerned with two of the most important but most difficult relationship issues—sexuality and communication. It also offers a brief commentary on cohabitation. Chapter 4 deals with issues that affect ongoing relationships, including relationship satisfaction, attributions and conflict, and social support. Taking into account the over-whelming social changes that have occurred in the past generation, Chapter 5 presents material on gender, power, and dual careers. Chapter 6 discusses relationship transformation, specifically divorce and remarriage. Finally, Chapter 7 presents some of the professional, ethical, and personal issues that confront couple therapists. Case examples are used in Chapters 2 through 7 to illustrate material.

Although the book is intended to communicate close relationships work to students and practitioners in psychology, counseling, marriage and family therapy, human services, and social work, it might also be of interest to advanced undergraduate students and to graduate students and professionals in these areas as well as those in sociology and communications. It could be used in both lecture and practicum courses.

I want to express my appreciation to the people who have had a part in this book. Close relationship scholars have provided valuable theory and research, and the many couples I have worked with showed me how this theory and research could be applied in therapy. I want to thank the wonderful professional staff at Brooks/Cole for their competent help. And Claire Verduin, humorous and patient as always, has once again been a wonderful editor. I would also like to thank the following reviewers, whose comments without question made this a better book: Joseph Brown, professor and director of the Family Therapy Program, Louisville, Kentucky; Stan Charnofsky, California State University—Northridge; Janine Roberts, University of Massachusetts; and Mark Wardon, Fairfield University.

Susan S. Hendrick

CHAPTER ONE

Close Relationships and Couple Counseling

Carol and Bob are a thirtyish couple seeking counseling. They have been married for five years, have one child, and are experiencing a growing distance between them, punctuated by disagreements.

ᵥᵥ

Daniel and Elena are in their mid-twenties and have been living together for about three years. Both have good jobs and are beginning to think about their future. They are seeking counseling because of increasing problems with intimacy, including sex.

ᵥᵥ

Joan and Kathy are a lesbian couple, around age 30, who have been intimate partners for seven years. Both are successful professionals. They have sought counseling because they have been experiencing increasing conflict, and Joan is afraid that Kathy is going to leave her.

ᵥᵥ

Chuck and Jennifer are in their early 40s, have been married for 20 years, and have two teenagers. They were referred for counseling by their family physician because they have been fighting in response to Jennifer's attempts to get Chuck more involved in family and household responsibilities.

ᵥᵥ

Bill and Todd, a gay male couple in their 30s, have been relationship partners for four years. Although they once shared many interests and activities, they have begun to pursue "separate" lives, and each partner is afraid that the other will have an affair. Thus they have sought counseling.

Close Relationships

These six couples have something in common—they are all involved in *close relationships*. They have something else in common—they are all seeking couple therapy. Couples such as these seek help from therapists every day, and it is such couples who prompted the current book, which is designed to introduce therapists and therapists-in-training to the developing literature on close, personal relationships.

What Is Close Relationships Research?

The multidisciplinary area of close relationships includes research from psychology, sociology, communications, family studies, and other disciplines and is concerned with interpersonal relationships that can be considered close or personal (for example, romantic relationships, friendships, workplace relationships). Close relationships research developed out of work on interpersonal attraction, courtship, marital satisfaction, and the like, but over the past decade it has come to occupy its own special niche in the literature. For the most part, the close relationships area has been confined to academic scholars from these various disciplines, and work has not been communicated to the larger world of practicing therapists. Yet virtually every concept and every research study in close relationships says something that is useful to therapists, particularly therapists who work with couples. To communicate that work is the goal of this book.

This book is not meant to provide an exhaustive review of the close relationships literature but rather to offer some representative theory and research useful to therapists and to invite further exploration of what close relationships has to offer the practitioner. Because the book is primarily concerned with presenting research and theory, it is not a therapy book per se. However, illustrations of couples and case examples from couple counseling are used to communicate the close relationships literature. The book is more about research than it is about therapy, but ultimately it is about both. The remainder of this chapter will focus on issues relevant to couple therapy. Subsequent chapters will focus on close relationships.

Introducing Couple Counseling

Imagine that the six couples introduced at the beginning of the chapter are new clients and that you have been the therapist assigned to work with them. What do you do first? What kinds of questions should you ask? What kinds of questions will they ask? What will they need from you, and what do you need to know?

These are the questions that every therapist, whether neophyte or seasoned professional, asks herself or himself when meeting new clients. And when working with a couple, the questions are multiplied by three, because there are somewhat different needs for each relationship partner and for the relationship itself.

Couple counseling involves a manageable complexity (at least numerically). It is more complex than individual work and simpler than family work, with the added advantage that the problems that need to be addressed are often right there in front of the therapist. Couples don't just talk about their problems, they display them. Partners sit close together or far apart. One partner orients to the other; the second partner orients to the therapist. They speak to each other, shout at each other, interrupt each other, ignore each other—all the while showing the therapist the "inside" of their relationship.

Sometimes couples profit from simply becoming aware of how they are behaving and what that behavior is communicating. In other situations, partners need a safe haven in which to put words to their behaviors. At still other times, partners know what they are saying and doing; they just need some strategies and support for saying and doing things differently. Whatever the reasons for seeking counseling, couples can be the most challenging, exciting, and rewarding of clients.

If couples range from adjusted and contented on one end to abusive and highly pathological on the other, then the couples discussed in this book are somewhere in the middle. They are not couples who are one step away from disaster. However, without timely and appropriate intervention, they might become so. Such couples are particularly appropriate for applying close relationships research, because this literature has emerged in large measure out of concerns about "normal" relationships—their processes and their problems. Relationships where abusive conflict, constant infidelity, or social class disadvantages are themes have not been a central part of close relationships work. This is beginning to change, and close relationships researchers are widening their lens, but in the meantime, a wealth of close relationships material exists that practicing therapists and therapists-in-training can use right now with moderately distressed couples.

Who Is a Couple?

Recent decades have brought about changes in our definition of a couple (Scanzoni, Polonko, Teachman, & Thompson, 1989). No longer do we assume that married, heterosexual partners are what we mean when we say *couple.* Today, cohabiting couples, premarital couples, lesbian couples, and gay male couples all join married couples in seeking help with their relationships.

If therapy is a continuum with individual treatment on one end and group treatment on the other, then couple treatment may be viewed as fitting between individual and family approaches. Individual-oriented therapists may view a couple as two individuals who are trying to work out their separate problems so as to be able to develop a healthy connection. Family-oriented therapists may see a couple as a subsystem of the family in which action in the subsystem inevitably produces reaction in the other parts of the system (and vice versa). A couple-oriented therapist acknowledges both the individuals and the larger family system but takes as the focus of interest the dyadic system—the two partners and the relationship between them.

Who Is the Client?

The treatment approach presented in the examples in this book is conjoint couple counseling in which both partners are seen together by one therapist. However, it is important to be aware that other treatment units may be appropriate in some situations. Baruth and Huber (1984) point out that the therapist needs to assess whether the partners' problems are really dyadic (in which case, couple counseling is indicated) or are more individual (perhaps indicating individual therapy for both partners). Variants of therapy include (1) individual therapy for each partner, with different therapists; (2) individual therapy for each partner, with the same therapist; (3) co-therapy, in which partners are seen together by two therapists; or (4) couples' group therapy, in which several couples are seen together, usually by one or two therapists (Baruth & Huber, 1984). In conjoint couple counseling, it is important to remember that there are really three clients: two partners and their relationship.

The Counseling Process

Although a substantial portion of virtually any type of counseling training is likely to be spent developing a particular theoretical orientation, much therapeutic work cuts across theory lines. Theoretical grounding will clearly influence the way in which a therapist fosters the therapeutic relationship (for example, psychoanalytic therapists may be less expressive than humanistic ones) or structures therapy (for example, behavioral therapists may be most likely to do formal assessment). However, issues of the therapeutic relationship and structuring the therapy are for the most part transtheoretical. Underlying the total process is the therapist's view of the world.

The Therapist's Worldview

The way in which a therapist views the world will to some extent drive therapy choices. A therapist who views human beings as proactive, naturally seeking growth and development, is likely to expect clients to be motivated and to give at least reasonably honest and self-disclosing answers in therapy. A comfortable therapy approach may be client-centered, with considerable give and take. On the other hand, the helping professional who sees human behavior as largely determined by early and often painful experiences may be less trusting of what is seen in therapy. The therapist may be less interactive and more observational with clients, quietly listening for what is "not said." A psychodynamic approach may be much more congruent with such a worldview. A professional's worldview is in process, just as is his or her therapy work. And it is important for the therapist to understand this perspective at any given point in time because it inevitably influences the conduct of therapy and the therapeutic relationship.

The Therapeutic Relationship

Whatever their theoretical orientation, most therapists recognize the fundamental importance of the relationship between therapist and client. Whether it is called the therapy relationship, the bond component of the working alliance (Safran & Segal, 1990), or something else, the quality of the bond between client and therapist is a major factor in successful psychotherapy. Safran and Segal (1990) discuss research indicating that therapist empathy is consistently related to positive therapy outcome (when assessed from the client's perspective). Qualities such as reciprocal affirmation between client and therapist are consistently predictive of outcome no matter who rates it. Conditions considered necessary for therapeutic change as set forth by Rogers (1992) include therapist genuineness (that is, congruency and integration within the therapy relationship); unconditional positive regard (that is, "prizing" the client); and empathy (that is, sensing the client's phenomenological experience "as if" it were the therapist's own). Thus, to establish the basic groundwork of the therapeutic relationship, a therapist tries to establish a basis of trust, create a setting of safety, model clear and nonjudgmental communication, build client self-esteem, and perform a number of other actions (Satir, 1967) that may vary depending on the therapist's theoretical orientation. Although these conditions may not always be sufficient for successful therapy outcome, it is difficult for more than symptom relief to occur without them.

The psychotherapy relationship has some properties in common with other close relationships. In fact, several scholars (Derlega, Hendrick, Winstead, & Berg, 1991) proposed that if "close relationships are those in which individuals have a strong impact on each other and influence each other frequently and in diverse ways and that tend to endure over some period of time," then "the therapy relationship is certainly a close relationship" (p. 3). The professional quality of the therapy relationship makes it different from other close relationships. However, factors that affect intimate relationships—attraction, communication, responsiveness, social support—are also relevant to the therapy relationship. Viewed from the close relationships perspective as well as from the traditional psychotherapy perspective, the client-therapist relationship is a unique and important one.

The therapist's relationship with a client couple is not only unique and important, it is also complicated. The therapist is the person who makes the couple dyad the therapy triad. The acceptance, valuing, and bonding between counselor and client described earlier has to be done "times two" in couple counseling. The therapist needs to appreciate each partner as both an individual and as part of the couple, understanding that a quality such as persistence, which may be adaptive and even admirable in an individual, can translate into stubbornness and an inability to compromise in couple interaction.

In working with an individual, a therapist has the luxury of "taking the client's side" for the most part. Couple counseling is different; on any issue, there are two sides—and maybe three. The therapist asks questions, listens to the clients tell their stories, and begins to "live with the couple in the triadic relationship," monitoring the therapist's responses to the clients, the clients' responses to the therapist, and the clients' responses to each other. Although it may appear that the couple therapist is not intitially "taking sides," the therapist is really siding with the relationship rather than with either partner in it. This does not mean, however, that the counselor never shows bias toward either partner; it simply means that the bias is directed fairly equally to both partners, insofar as that is possible.

For example, in a session with a married couple in which the wife is being exceedingly demanding and inflexible about an issue, the therapist may underscore her negativity, seeming to "side" with the husband. However, later when the wife is asking (rather than demanding) some clear communication with the husband (who is hedging, as usual), the therapist may support the wife's requests for communication and underscore the husband's vagueness, thereby seeming to "side" with the wife. Most couples bring a problematic system to the therapist—a system to which both partners contribute. It is rare to find a relationship in which both partners cannot be supported—and confronted—by the therapist.

In addition to fairness, a couple therapist needs to be a careful observer of nonverbal behavior—what people *do* as well as what they *say*. A sense of humor and an awareness of the frailty of the human condition are also helpful, if not essential. A couple therapist needs to have the qualities that contribute to the therapeutic bond, as discussed earlier, and also needs to be able to focus on client feelings and target interventions appropriately (Orlinsky & Howard, 1986). Ideally, specific therapy skills are augmented by a curiosity about, a respect for, and even a delight in the partnered intimate relationship.

Structuring Therapy

Although the flow of couple therapy has a great deal to do with the clients themselves, the therapist needs to structure initial data-gathering and set a tone of hopefulness in the early sessions. One possible approach to structuring therapy has been adapted to couples and is shown in Box 1.1.

BOX 1.1
Format for Structuring Early Therapy Sessions

Session I
1. Get demographic information (including referral source) on an intake form. Are there any other significant people involved (for example, extended family) in the decision to seek treatment? Is any feedback needed to referral source?
2. Get clients' perceptions of the presenting issues. Why are they seeking help? What are their goals and expectations for treatment?
3. Why now? What specific circumstances prompted the couple to seek therapy at this time? Get specific details of the relevant persons involved, specific symptoms, and increasing or decreasing severity and length of symptoms.
4. To the extent possible, get a brief description of the clients' current life including relationship, employment, and so on.
5. Prepare the couple for therapy. Explain how therapy might be helpful. Explain the therapy process (for example, client's role, therapist's role, confidentiality and its limits, appointments and payment). Restate any goals that they have given and note that more specific goals may be spelled out after a couple of sessions. Inform the clients that the next session or two will be devoted to history-taking. Have release forms signed if indicated. (If needed, assessment for substance abuse, violence, suicide, and major mental disorder may also be part of this initial intake procedure.)

Session II
1. Assuming that partners are being seen together and that individual psychosocial histories are being taken, briefly check in about the clients' welfare during the intervening period.
2. Get a family history, including members of family of origin, relational quality, major life events, and description of parents and siblings. What was it like growing up in that family?

   Solicit information regarding the client's social history, including friends and companions, history of relationships, degree of disclosure in relationships, fears and expectations regarding relationships, and other life experiences. Include school experiences and employment history.

   Get medical history, including major illnesses and hospitalizations, current medications, previous psychological treatment, and any other family illnesses (for example, parent or child) that have an impact on the client's life.
3. If possible, try to summarize the major themes brought out in the history.

GO THROUGH STEPS 2 AND 3 WITH THE OTHER PARTNER.

4. Finally, get a history of the partners' relationship, including when and how they met, what attracted them to each other, and how the relationship has proceeded. Be aware of how the story is told as well as what is contained in the story.

After session II
1. Give an initial diagnostic impression, including a formal diagnosis and the reasons for it.
2. Give a prognostic impression and the reasons for it.
3. Develop an initial treatment plan. Such a plan might include communications training, cognitive-behavioral strategies to limit conflict, and stress-reduction techniques such as relaxation. The plan might call for eventual referral to a couples therapy group.

Session III
1. Present treatment plan to the couple and get their input. Revise plan as needed. Begin work (noting that, in fact, work began when the therapist and the couple first met).

Session I is incredibly important. If some connection between therapist and clients can be made, then therapy can proceed; if not, the work may be over before it starts. The therapist should display warmth, make eye contact with each partner, and in general "welcome" the pair into therapy. One partner will typically have made the appointment, so care must be given to bringing the other partner into the context. Even if the telephoning partner has had no personal contact with the therapist, the other partner may be somewhat wary of starting "one down" and should be given some extra attention.

The interpersonal aspects of the first session are important; however, much practical work also takes place. Securing basic demographic information, then finding out why the clients are seeking therapy, and "why now?" can occupy 5 minutes or 50 minutes, depending on the situation. The clients may begin "telling their story," at least in part, but complete history-taking will likely have to wait until the next session. The first session can be structured rather precisely in small "blocks" of time devoted to introductions, identifying the problem, observing client behaviors, and so on (for a step-by-step guide, see Goldenberg & Goldenberg, 1990), or it can be approached more as a series of larger stages (for example, a social stage, a problem stage; see Haley, 1987). Whatever the approach, the session should probably conclude with some goal-setting and agreement for how treatment will proceed.

Session II is likely to involve taking a psychosocial history from one or both partners. One approach is to see both partners together for the first session, then see each partner individually to get their histories, and then bring them back together for the rest of the therapy work. This approach has the advantage of allowing the therapist to establish a "personal" relationship with each partner while getting the histories in more detail. One disadvantage is that partners may be inclined to tell the therapist "secrets" that they want to be kept from the other partner. Still another approach is to have the partners together at all sessions but to get individual histories as well as a joint history. An advantage to this approach is that it allows each partner to eavesdrop on the other partner's description of his or her background. Even though the information is likely to have been heard before, there can be a new "aha" experience as one partner hears again that the other was demeaned as a child and had very low self-esteem. Realizing once again that the partner's current difficulties in handling criticism may stem directly from childhood experiences does not necessarily make the current situation any less frustrating, but it can help the listener take things less personally and be at least temporarily more patient with the partner. And a temporary "cease-fire" may allow enough space for initiation of the therapeutic work. After getting detailed information from the individual partners, it is important to obtain a joint history from the couple.

These earliest sessions are used to gather many different kinds of information. For example, the therapist can see how partners communicate with each other and with the therapist. Both verbal and nonverbal behaviors are richly informative. Questions such as, How did you meet? What attracted you to each other? and What do you want to happen to your relationship? are all valuable (Lukas, 1993). Noting what evokes emotion, what sparks conflict, and what creates distance is as much a part of data-gathering as is taking a psychosocial history or giving an assessment instrument.

Perhaps after the first session, but surely after two or three sessions, a treatment strategy can be developed. Depending on a therapist's theoretical orientation and the couple's presenting issues, partners may participate in a variety of kinds of assessment. Completion of measures of relationship satisfaction (including sexual satisfaction), conflict, depression, and so on might be sought by a behavioral therapist (see Dattilio & Padesky, 1990). A systems-oriented therapist might want a genogram (pictorial family tree), or a psychoanalytic therapist might want partners to take various projective measures. A useful measure for relatively "healthy" relationship partners is the Myers-Briggs Type Indicator (MBTI) (see Myers & McCaulley, 1985), which can help partners understand how they are similar and different without either partner being the identified patient.

Difficult Issues in Assessing a Couple

Couple therapy is challenging, even under ideal circumstances, but particular issues such as infidelity, substance abuse, or violence may greatly complicate the process and may even be considered crisis situations. As Dattilio & Padesky (1990) have said, "Crises such as these usually warrant emergency intervention, sometimes over several sessions. Diffusing the emergency typically takes precedence over the normal course of intake" (p. 83). (See also Jacobson & Gurman, 1986; and Dattilio & Padesky, 1990; for a full discussion of special issues.)

Although infidelity is typically thought of as sexual involvement outside marriage, it is used here to refer to sexual involvement outside any partnered romantic relationship. Such involvement may satisfy an individual partner's needs (assuage loneliness, affirm attractiveness) or may fulfill some purpose for the relationship (getting the partner's attention, evoking jealousy). It may be a signal from one partner to the other to "pay attention before it's too late." However, before the meaning of the infidelity can be explored, both partners must become aware of the behavior. It is not wise for a therapist to keep secrets about a partner's infidelity, though such situations do sometimes occur. (Confidentiality issues are discussed in Chapter 7.) One approach is to tell partners that therapy can only be truly effective if partners are honest with one another and "put all their cards on the table." In addition, current concerns about AIDS raise ethical questions if one partner is having an affair (see Chapter 7). In fact, when couple therapy seems to be "stuck" for no reason, it may imply that one partner has an extra-relationship involvement. Of course, it is extremely important to assess whether or not infidelity is a problem in the relationship. Some couples may have agreed that their relationship is sexually nonexclusive (Constantine, 1986), and infidelity may not be the problem that has brought them into treatment.

Another critical area of assessment is substance abuse. Substance abuse is connected with numerous problems, including suicide, homicide, and abuse of adults and children (Lukas, 1993), so assessing for it is imperative. Lukas suggests that the therapist always ask about substance use and abuse. The initial questions can be embedded in a medical history and might refer to such things as substances, quantity, frequency of use, previous attempts to stop, and so on. Exploration of substance abuse in a couple situation may be done jointly or separately and may depend on whether abuse has been identified as part of the presenting problem. Interventions for dealing with the abuse will vary depending on whether it is past or ongoing, whether mild or severe, whether covertly or overtly part of the couple's presenting problem, and so on. If "recovery" is part of the agreed-upon therapy agenda, then therapy may consist of both abuse-focused and relationship-focused interventions (O'Farrell, 1986), and outside entities such as Alcoholics Anonymous (AA) or Narcotics Anonymous (NA) may become part of the treatment. Substance abuse is a common and extremely intractable problem, and to deal with it well, therapists need considerable training and experience.[*]

Another difficult and all too frequent occurrence is relationship violence. Violence may be directed at either persons or property, but abuse is typically person-directed and usually goes from man to woman. Some issues about abuse are discussed in later chapters; the focus here is on initial assessment of violence. Marital violence (or, more generally, relationship violence) may consist of physical violence, sexual violence, psychological abuse, and violence to pets and property (Rosenbaum & O'Leary, 1986). Alcohol use is frequently associated with violence, as are drug abuse, gambling, and similar addictive behaviors. If violence or abuse is suspected, Rosenbaum and O'Leary recommend making individual interviews a routine part of a couple's intake assessment. If it is determined that a female partner (or one or both partners in a same-sex couple) feels in immediate danger,

---

[*]Information about education and training relevant to substance abuse may be obtained from the National Association of Alcohol and Drug Abuse Counselors (NAADAC), 3717 Columbia Pike, Suite 300, Arlington, VA 22204.

then that person's safety becomes top priority. Referral to a shelter and facilitation of legal remedies may be required (Rosenbaum & O'Leary, 1986). The violence must stop. Then decisions can be made as to whether and how to work with a couple.

Cognitive-behavioral approaches may be particularly useful in violence situations (Dattilio & Padesky, 1990; Rosenbaum & O'Leary, 1986). (For an assessment protocol to be used where abuse is suspected, see Lukas, 1993.) It is important for a therapist to become familiar both with the general literature available on assessment and treatment of relationship violence and with the relevant specific policies in a given work setting and the legal requirements in the therapist's area of residence.

Although issues of infidelity, substance abuse, and violence are serious special concerns in couple counseling, there are many other possible issues such as suicide potential (Lukas, 1993), eating disorders (Foster, 1986), and the like. Readers are referred to the extensive and specialized literatures available in these areas.

Approaches to Couple Counseling

The choices that a therapist makes about handling special problems as well as routine issues in couple counseling are linked directly to the therapist's guiding theoretical approach to the therapy. This discussion is designed to be applicable to therapists from virtually every theoretical orientation. This is particularly appropriate because the close relationships literature itself reflects a variety of theoretical approaches. But to provide a context, the next section will present a brief overview of the major theoretical systems applied to couples work, concluding with the approach underlying the applied examples presented here.

Psychoanalytic Approach

Psychoanalytic theory, beginning with Freud, has been perhaps the most influential of the theoretical systems used in therapy. Basic psychoanalytic concepts applied to couple therapy have been summarized by Baruth and Huber (1984) as follows:

1. Unconscious internal conflicts of one or both partners cause marital problems.
2. The unconscious must be made conscious in order to resolve conflicts.

3. Verbalizations that follow one another in therapy are connected, either consciously or unconsciously.
4. Emotional insight must come before behavior change.
5. Transference and countertransference issues occur in therapy.

If these are a therapist's operating assumptions in therapy, then family of origin issues, relationship history, and current relationship functioning are likely to be analyzed in terms of their genetic origins. In fact, "individual psychodynamics are postulated as structuring the marital relationship by unconscious family-of-origin motivations of the transference-like qualities" (Dare, 1986, p. 26). However, although these therapist conceptualizations may be relatively "pure," the nondirective, interpretive stance of the psychoanalytic therapist is likely to be modified in conjoint therapy where some measure of directiveness may be necessary (Dare, 1986). Thus, techniques such as interpretation, the analysis of resistance, and dreamwork may be supplemented by behavioral strategies such as contracting.

Cognitive-Behavioral Approach

The cognitive-behavioral perspective as framed here encompasses cognitive and behavioral approaches to couple treatment. This perspective characterizes behavior as a product of both the social environment and cognitive-perceptual processes (Jacobson & Holtzworth-Munroe, 1986). This approach does not focus on the genetic origins of behavior but rather works at changing behaviors that are contributing to couple dysfunction. Ideas that might be loosely considered "tenets" of this approach are:

- Treatment should involve an analysis of what caused the relationship dysfunction and what is maintaining it.
- Partners need to learn to emphasize the positives and strengths in the relationship.
- Partners need to learn to appreciate and reward positives rather than to punish negatives.
- Partners need to be mutually rewarding.
- Relationship skills can be learned.

The cognitive-behavioral approach involves a focus on overt behavior, an analysis of the presenting problem, and formulation (and later assessment) of a specific treatment program (Baruth & Huber, 1984). The couple therapist employing this overall approach is likely to use techniques for increasing positive partner exchanges, improving both communication and problem-solving skills, helping partners learn to accept responsibility for behaviors, and other interventions (Jacobson & Holtzworth-Munroe, 1986).

In addition, although the therapist's role has been rather directive and with an emphasis on objectivity (the assessment-treatment-evaluation process), more recently the therapy relationship has received increasing emphasis (Safran & Segal, 1990). (For a clear description of couples cognitive therapy, see Dattilio & Padesky, 1990.)

Systems Approach

The breadth of the theoretical models within the systems framework is exciting and sometimes confusing for the beginning therapist. Included in these are the strategic approaches of Haley (1987) and others such as the Milan group (Selvini Palazzoli, Boscolo, Cecchin, & Prata, 1978), the structural approach of Minuchin (1974; Minuchin & Nichols, 1993), Bowen's more dynamic work (1978), Satir's communication orientation (1967; Satir & Baldwin, 1983), and others. Systems theorists, broadly construed, are likely to view a couple relationship, especially a marital one, as a fairly stable interactional system (Todd, 1986). A couple seeks therapy when that system becomes unstable or stable but unsatisfactory. Basic tenets of the systems approach vary depending on the therapist's vantage point, but according to Worden (1994) and other scholars, the systems approach may include these tenets:

- Partners need to settle issues between them rather than pulling in another family member as confidant or scapegoat.
- Boundaries between family members and generational systems (that is, children, parents, grandparents) should be flexible so that people are neither too enmeshed nor too distant.
- Power in the family is the ability to influence another, it has both overt and covert qualities, and it can be harnessed productively.
- Intimacy is important for everyone, and there are many positive ways in which it can work for a couple and in a family.
- Communication is extremely important; improved communication is essential for other positive changes to occur.

Each model of systems therapy is oriented somewhat differently; however, some of the undergirding assumptions about the system and the change process for the system are shared. The process of therapy may involve many different interventions, ranging from the use of a genogram, to tasks to be performed outside therapy, to bringing the partners' extended families into therapy. The therapy relationship has always been considered important, with the therapist needing to "join" the family as a trusted person. Depending on the approach chosen, the therapist may become almost a family member—or may remain a somewhat more objective consultant.

(For a detailed description of various systems approaches, see Becvar & Becvar, 1988; for guidelines to interviewing, see Worden, 1994.)

The Communication Approach

Although this book is meant to be transtheoretical and to communicate close relationships research to the practitioner, nevertheless, there is substantial applied material in the text, primarily in the form of case examples that conclude Chapters 2 through 7. These case examples illustrate close relationships theory and research, yet they are written on the basis of certain therapeutic assumptions and a definite therapist orientation. The assumptions and the orientation are drawn directly from the communications work of Satir (1967; Satir & Baldwin, 1983), mentioned earlier under systems approaches. This approach stems from the idea that people inevitably communicate, and they communicate most effectively when they communicate clearly and openly. As Satir (1967) noted, "As a therapist, I have found that the more covertly and indirectly people communicate, the more dysfunctional they are likely to be" (p. 17). Although this approach does not assume that communication is *all* there is to interpersonal relating, communication is viewed as having central importance. Some additional assumptions are:

- A relationship partner may know what their partner *says*, but they should not assume that they know what the partner *means*.
- If there is any question about a communication, it is important to ask for clarification. It is also important that partners be willing and able to clarify their own communications to each other.
- Mind reading in relationships does not work.
- Functional communicators send complete and clear messages and do not overgeneralize.
- Partners need to be able to ask for what they want in the relationship. Asking does not assure getting, but not asking assures not getting.
- Relationships require negotiation; negotiation requires good communication.

The therapist working from the communications perspective will first observe a couple's verbal and nonverbal communication style and then seek to modify it by (1) modeling clear communication, (2) seeking clarification frequently, (3) commenting on what the therapist sees and hears (for example, "When Mary starts talking about the conflict at home, John closes his eyes and looks bored"), and (4) in general raising the partners' awareness about their communication patterns. Although the therapist may initially serve as a sort of "translator" for the couple, the ultimate goal is to increase communication competence. Specific training in communication skills (see Chapter 3) is part of this therapy approach.

I have touched on three of the major psychotherapy approaches, explaining how they might be applied to couple counseling and discussing the communications approach employed in the case examples in this book. There are undoubtedly as many models for couple counseling as there are therapy models in general. Thus, whether a therapist practices Eclectic, Adlerian, Rational-Emotive, Reality, Transactional Analysis, Gestalt, Humanistic/Existential, or some other form of therapy, the work is applicable to couples.

Looking Ahead

The following chapters in this book will cover aspects of relationship initiation and development, relationship maintenance, and relationship dissolution. This includes close relationship research on interpersonal attraction, relationship development, and love that has applications to couple counseling. Discussions of sexuality, communication, social support, and other topics follow. The overwhelming social changes that have affected contemporary relationships—particularly gender roles and dual careers—are considered next. Finally, some of the professional, ethical, and personal issues that confront couple therapists are presented.

Summary

Close relationships research has grown over the past decade and is directly applicable to therapy with couples. The therapist's view of the world has a considerable impact on all facets of the therapy process, including the therapist-client relationship. The therapy relationship is based on mutual respect, trust, and valuing, which allows the client a safe forum in which to do the work of therapy. In many ways, the therapy relationship qualifies as a "close" relationship. Couple counseling involves a process of rapport-building, data-gathering, and ongoing therapy work. Couple crisis problems such as infidelity, substance abuse, and relationship violence all increase the complexity of couple counseling. Some of the prevailing theoretical perspectives that have been applied effectively to couple counseling include psychoanalytic, cognitive-behavioral, and systems approaches, with the communications approach most evident here. Pragmatism, humor, and flexibility are also helpful to a therapist when undertaking the interesting and complex task of couple counseling.

CHAPTER TWO

Attraction, Courtship, and Love

I'll never forget the first time I saw her. We were at a party, and some mutual friends introduced us. I felt like there were sparks between us. She's tall and dark-haired, the type of woman I have always been attracted to. I wanted to know everything about her immediately, and I guess she felt the same way. We left the party and went out for coffee. We stayed up all night talking about everything in the world—our families, our work, our religious beliefs, our favorite flavor of ice cream—just everything. We saw each other the following night and have been together ever since.

&⟂

Romantic relationships begin in many different ways. One person may choose the other person as a partner, or the choosing may be mutual. There may be an actual decision to have a relationship, or two people may just seem to wander into the relationship. Although therapists spend time working on their own intimate relationships as well as aiding clients in working out problems in close relationships, helping professionals are often given very little detailed scientific information about how or why relationships begin and develop. Everyone has some general notions about how people get together—college students meet each other in class; working people meet each other in the office or factory. In addition, formal knowledge on courtship and mate selection is available from social science research.

Choosing a Partner

Human beings are essentially a social species, so finding a relationship partner is an important life task. Some people "go through" a number of relationships before finding someone to share a life with; others commit themselves to the first person they date. Today, young adults in the United

States are taking more time with this process. People are waiting longer to get married, and the age of first marriage for women and men is higher than it has been in decades, about 24 years for women and 26 years for men (Surra, 1990). It would be ideal if this trend indicated that people are waiting to marry because they are making more mature relationship choices, but that may only be wishful thinking. Factors such as cohabitation (which allows marital deferral) and economic stress (which may require marital deferral) are likely reasons for the increase in age at first marriage. In the process of actually selecting or finding a partner, a number of variables are important. These variables include similarity, self-disclosure, and physical attractiveness.

Similarity

One of the most compelling bases for attraction appears to be similarity, whether similarity of attitudes (Byrne, 1971), personality characteristics (for example, Lloyd, Paulsen, & Brockner, 1983), economic characteristics (Byrne, Clore, & Worchel, 1966), or other factors. People seem to be more easily attracted to others who are similar—and to be more likely to marry such people. *Homogamy*, or the tendency to choose a mate similar to oneself, continues to be the norm for marital choice (Surra, 1990), at least for such aspects of life as religion, race/ethnicity, language, education, and for the most part age. However, *heterogamy*, mating with someone different from oneself, is becoming more common. Heterogamy is more likely among younger people and will probably increase as people widen their social networks in our increasingly global society. For example, Tucker and Mitchell-Kernan (1990) found that interracial marriage occurred more frequently when persons moved away from "home" into communities with greater tolerance for such relationships. Getting away from family and social networks may free people to experience new attitudes and behaviors. The opposite can also occur. Recently a young wife said, "I met my husband on the east coast while he was in the Navy. We met, got married, and lived in the east until he got out of the service; then we went back to his hometown in Texas to live. Well, he put on his jeans and cowboy boots and hat—and all the attitudes that went with them. The man I had married just 'disappeared.'" Although some scholars propose that complementarity (the notion that "opposites attract") may also be a factor in attraction and relationship well-being (for example, Winch, 1958), similarity is viewed as the stronger positive force. When counseling a couple, emphasizing and strengthening partner similarities is one useful strategy.

For example, it might be helpful for the couple just mentioned to explore both the things that have stayed the same during their transition from east to west and the things that have changed. Perhaps the husband just takes for granted that donning his old cowboy boots and cowboy hat means taking on his old attitudes. Or perhaps he doesn't. It is possible that because he looks different his wife assumes that he is different.

Having similar attitudes and backgrounds may be important in finding the right partner, but these factors are "givens"; they don't have much to do with the interactions that occur between two people. One aspect of such interaction is communication, specifically self-disclosure.

Self-Disclosure

Self-disclosure refers to a willingness to tell another person honestly what one is thinking or feeling. It means taking off the social mask of a prescribed role and revealing oneself to another. However, self-disclosure is a complicated phenomenon, and more is not necessarily better. First explored by Jourard (1964), self-disclosure research has been concerned with such things as reciprocity of disclosure and whether it is better to disclose a lot or a little information. Most recently, Derlega and his colleagues (Derlega, Metts, Petronio, & Margulis, 1993) have discussed self-disclosure in great depth, showing how disclosure can transform a close relationship by making it more intimate even as the disclosure itself is transformed by the relationship. For example, as the relationship reaches a deep level of intimacy, the rate of self-disclosure may slow down.

Men and women appear to differ in self-disclosure, with women typically disclosing more. However, much has to do with what the disclosure is about and how it is measured (Hill & Stull, 1987). Derlega and colleagues (1993) conjecture that women and men grow up in essentially different subcultures in the Western world. Women grow up learning that it is good to be nurturant, acceptable to be vulnerable, and that communication is a good way to connect with others. Men, on the other hand, often grow up learning that it is good to be successful, acceptable to be aggressive, and that connecting with others (except sexually) is a secondary consideration (Gilbert, 1993).

Traditional sex roles, partitioning women and men into the areas of intimacy and achievement, respectively, have inevitably influenced how, when, and how much men and women disclose to their partners. Of course, there is much overlap in women's and men's disclosure patterns, but it is the differences that tend to disrupt relationships and propel couples into counseling. For example, partners may have solid communication, except at the times when one partner (the woman) gets angry and the other partner (the man) withdraws into silence. A therapist can help the couple appreciate their communication strengths and then begin to work on the problem areas. Explaining to clients that women and men grow up with some differences in communication styles and skills may help partners take their problems a bit less personally.

Physical Attractiveness

People depend on visual cues to tell them about the world; how something looks is important. How a person looks is important, too, and research indicates that physical attractiveness in a partner is significant. Fortunately, as the old saying goes, "beauty is in the eye of the beholder"; different physical qualities are considered attractive by different people.

Research has also been done on the matching hypothesis, which essentially says that people of a certain level of physical attractiveness will seek relationship partners who are at the same level. Empirical support for the matching hypothesis has been mixed for dating couples (Berscheid, Dion, Walster, & Walster, 1971), though other research with married couples found that partners were somewhat matched on attractiveness (Murstein & Christy, 1976). In a meta-analysis of attractiveness studies, Feingold (1988) found modest correlations between relationship partners on physical attractiveness and conjectured that physical attractiveness may be most important at the beginning of a relationship as a kind of "screening device" but may become less so as the relationship progresses. Research by Nevid (1984) is consistent with this theory. Although men were more likely than were women to seek attractive dating partners (particularly when the relationship was to be a sexual one), when considering long-term partners, both women and men focused less on physical qualities and more on such things as honesty.

Physical attractiveness in clients is not typically thought about a great deal, and its absence may be more important than its presence. For example, because of what we know about societal pressure for attractiveness, as well as the research literature on attractiveness, relationship partners might be expected to look fairly similar in terms of both physical characteristics and standards of grooming. If that is not the case, if partners differ greatly in these dimensions, it is useful information for the therapist. Attractiveness issues may not be the presenting problem for such a couple, but they are likely to fit in somewhere.

Additional Influences

There are many additional influences on how relationships develop. It is not surprising that people like others with good looks, intelligence, a pleasant personality, and so on. But it may be a surprise to some that people who are "perfect" are not as well liked as those who have a flaw or two (Aronson,

Willerman, & Floyd, 1966). People seem to want their significant others to be good—but not perfect. Being valued by another person is also important; in fact, one study found that people who believed their partner had positive characteristics *and* that the partner liked them were more likely to fall in love (Aron, Dutton, Aron, & Iverson, 1989).

Additional influences on relationship development may include individual factors such as personality style (whether someone is outgoing or shy), relationship factors such as whether partners find the relationship rewarding (Rusbult, Johnson, & Morrow, 1986), and social network factors such as opposition to the relationship (Surra, 1987). Although not all of these factors can be discussed, it is essential to recognize their existence and the complexity of the relationship-building process. The next section considers several theories concerned with how relationships develop once two people have gotten together.

Models of Relationship Development

In a review of the courtship literature, Cate and Lloyd (1988) divided the theories illustrating premarital relationship establishment into three categories: (1) compatibility, (2) interpersonal process, and (3) exchange theories.

Compatibility

One area of compatibility relates to partner similarity and complementarity discussed earlier. Another approach, stimulus-value-role theory (Murstein, 1976), is considered more of a stage theory wherein different characteristics are important to partners at different points in the development of the relationship. With this perspective, surface characteristics such as physical attractiveness might be more important early in the relationship, values more important later, and successfully negotiating gender role issues important still later. For example, David and Maria were strongly physically attracted to each other. It was not until they had dated a few times that they discussed their religious, political, and social attitudes. And not until they had been together for several months did they work out issues about balancing time with each other, time alone, and time with friends.

Interpersonal Process

Close relationship researchers like Duck and Sants (1983) have increasingly recognized the "complex interplay of courtship partners with each other, as well as their individual and joint interaction with their extended family, their social networks, and their larger social and physical environment" (Hendrick & Hendrick, 1992a, p. 151). One interpersonal approach involves studying the "pathways" that various couples take toward marriage (Cate, Huston, & Nesselroade, 1986; Lloyd & Cate, 1985). Based on many couples' descriptions of the various ups and downs and turning points in their relationships, it appears that some couples get involved very quickly (accelerated development), some progress slowly and painfully (prolonged development), and some move at a moderate pace and appear to have the fewest problems (intermediate development). Interpersonal process research is characterized by its focus on the dynamic, changeable aspects of a relationship rather than on the relatively static aspects (such as religious preference) that have previously received so much attention.

Exchange Theories

Exchange theorists use the words *rewards* and *costs*, analyzing relationships as if they were business transactions. Rusbult (1983; Rusbult et al., 1986) developed a model of relationship investment based on exchange precepts. The model proposes, first, that relationship satisfaction is greater when individuals believe they are receiving greater rewards and incurring fewer costs in the relationship than they deserve. And second, commitment increases along with increases in satisfaction, and in resource investment (for example, emotional or financial resources) and with decreases in the acceptability of relationship alternatives (that is, other partners or the option of being without a partner). Not surprisingly, in relevant research, most of this model appears to "work." Indeed, people who feel more rewarded in their close relationships are more invested in and satisfied with them, and commitment increases as the viability of alternative partners decreases (Surra, 1990). Costs, however, do not seem as predictive of relationship quality. Using the example of Maria and David, both partners give a lot of time and energy to each other and to the relationship (resource investment), both enjoy the relationship (feel rewarded) and are satisfied with it, and both are becoming increasingly committed. In addition, neither one even considers dating anyone else (decreasing relationship alternatives).

Equity theory, an extension of exchange theory (Walster, Berscheid, & Walster, 1973, 1976), reaffirms that people like fairness or equitable treatment in a relationship, and if one partner is greatly under- or over-benefited relative to the other partner, she or he will try to restore an equitable balance. For example, Maria recently lost her job, so David has been paying for all their expenses. However, as soon as she finds a new job, Maria intends to again pay her "fair share."

People typically do not like to talk about intimate relationships in economic terms; however, this approach is one sensible way to view the balance of positives and negatives that partners experience. Couples seeking relationship counseling are often experiencing an imbalance. One partner may feel more rewarded than the other. The partner initiating therapy is usually the one who feels less rewarded. More commonly, however, one or both partners feel that their rewards have decreased, their costs have increased, and the relationship just isn't much fun anymore.

While I have described these three approaches to relationships as though they were mutually exclusive, in fact, they all contribute to progression in a relationship. When two people first meet, it is likely that compatibility of interests, backgrounds, and individual characteristics such as physical attractiveness are important in getting the relationship off to a good start. As the relationship continues, interpersonal interactions (including everything from communication to critical events) are likely to determine progress or decline. Often, a relationship must continue for some time before the partners develop a good idea not only of the relative rewards and costs of the relationship but also of the relative balance of rewards and costs between the partners. One factor that helps closeness develop in a relationship is trust.

Trust is an important factor in relationships. As Holmes and Rempel (1989) note, "issues of trust have their origins in the dialectic between people's hopes and fears as close relationships develop" (p. 187). Individuals typically have both approach and avoidance tendencies when it comes to close relationships. As they become closer to one another, they typically become more dependent on the other person as well as more vulnerable to them. And vulnerability can be scary.

Trust seems to be both an intrapersonal and an interpersonal phenomenon (Holmes & Rempel, 1989). An individual may have a natural inclination to be trusting or mistrusting of others; that is the intrapersonal part. In a particular relationship, that same individual may be more or less trusting of the relationship partner. That is the interpersonal part. To use the previous example, for David to develop trust in Maria, he needs to feel that he is special to her and that she will do whatever she can to aid him, sometimes even putting his welfare above her own. It takes time and consistency of behavior to build trust. Holmes and Rempel (1989) propose that relationship partners who are high in trust are not unaware of each other's faults but rather tend to give each other the benefit of the doubt because there is an overall context of trust. On the other hand, low trust relationship partners are more likely to "keep score" and to let any negative interactions outweigh positive ones. If a therapist is counseling a couple in a developing relationship, it may be important to assess each individual's tendency to be trusting or mistrusting as well as the trust issues the couple is negotiating. Of course, partners who are high in trust and who give each other the benefit of the doubt are less likely to be seen in therapy.

Although trust is important to relationship development, it is not necessarily the first characteristic thought of when one is asked to name the necessary conditions for a successful romantic relationship. The characteristic most likely to be mentioned first is *love* (Simpson, Campbell, & Berscheid, 1986).

All About Love

Love may be the single most powerful element in a close relationship. It influences other elements, such as self-disclosure, and is in turn influenced by them. It is frequently ignored by therapists counseling couples, except to the extent that partners either do or do not love each other enough to work on their relationship. Being attuned to the more subtle aspects of love can be important in couple counseling. Love is of central importance to intimate relationships, and the relationship literature has a great deal to offer on the topic.

Love is a term of endearment upon which people put heavy demands. It is expected to describe affection between parent and child, between lover and lover, and even between friends. Whether it refers to a partner or to a favorite flavor of ice cream, the word (if not the behavior) is the same. Although many types of love are grist for the counselor's therapeutic mill, romantic love is most relevant to couple counseling, and there is considerable recent theory and research on the topic.

History of Love

Romantic love has been around for a long time, but only in the 20th century has it become inextricably linked to marriage. Zick Rubin (1970, 1973) was a social science pioneer in the study of loving and liking. Early on, love was categorized into two major types: passionate and companionate (Berscheid & Walster, 1978; Walster & Walster, 1978). If passionate love is like a roaring fire, then companionate love is the glowing embers that remain after the fire has burned down. Although considerable research on love has occurred since these concepts were introduced (for example, Davis & Todd, 1982; Fehr, 1988; Hazan & Shaver, 1987; Sternberg, 1986, 1987), the concepts are very resilient. Many people still believe that only two (or at least very few) types of love exist.

Love Styles

Sociologist John Alan Lee was an exception. Lee did extensive reading and research on love and, after interviewing hundreds of people, developed a multidimensional theory of love (1973). These dimensions can be referred to as *love styles*. Although these love styles are not mutually exclusive—indeed, every person has aspects of nearly all of them—it is useful to think about these ideal types when we talk about love. The six major dimensions or styles of love, described in detail below, include: eros, ludus, storge, pragma, mania, and agape.

EROS is a love style reflecting passionate intensity and wholehearted involvement. An eros lover has definite physical preferences in a partner (for example, blond or dark, blue- or brown-eyed, tall or short) and may react strongly to physical form. Love at first sight is a definite possibility for this love style, and this immediate intensity is reflected in a wish to communicate fully and to quickly become emotionally and physically involved. There is eagerness to be with the partner and a wish for openness, honesty, and sincerity. The erotic lover wants the relationship to develop mutually but does not demand mutuality from the partner. Although an erotic lover relates with focused intensity, he or she is not possessive or jealous. The passage that opened this chapter describes an eros relationship.

LUDUS is a love style based on the courtly tradition of love as a game. It is a playful and nonserious style characterized by wanting to have a good time and avoid being tied down. A ludus lover has no one preferred physical type, so the field of potential partners is broad. A ludic lover avoids deep emotional commitments and will not spend too much time with any one partner. The ludic person will be wary of any partner who becomes too involved and will try to help the partner regain some distance and perspective. Although love is a game, it is one to be played for mutual enjoyment, so it is not in anyone's best interests for feelings to get hurt. Insincerity and nondisclosure are justified as part of the "rules of the game," but there is no desire to inflict pain. (It is likely that someone who enjoys inflicting pain on a partner is dysfunctional rather than ludic.) A ludic lover enjoys sex and variety in sexual activity, but sex is a recreational activity rather than a means of communication. Ludic love is best played with several partners, preferably all ludic.

STORGE refers to love based on friendship. Although it is rarely the basis for poetry or romantic novels, nevertheless it is love that lasts. Storgic love develops slowly over time, without either eros's desire for immediate closeness or ludus's desire for distance. Storge requires a sharing of attitudes and values, gradual development of intimacy and trust, and an ability to be each other's "best friend" in addition to best lover. There is no preferred physical type, and sexuality is something to be gradually incorporated into the relationship, often not until the relationship has endured for some time. The relationship is generally relaxed, without the need to control strong emotions. Storgic lovers are loyal and patient; they are willing to wait for what they want.

PRAGMA is just like it sounds, pragmatic and practical. This is love that has a clear notion of what would be desirable in a partner and then goes looking for those qualities. A matchmaker or computer dating service might give pragmatic lovers the kind of predictability they seek. The pragmatic love style is looking for contentment and a mate with whom she or he is compatible. Pragma will look for similarity in a partner (unless complementarity on certain qualities is desired) and will avoid emotional extremes. The whole process of getting to know a partner and developing a relationship requires rationality and patience. Sexual satisfaction is viewed as only one of several important relationship components. A pragmatic lover knows that a suitable mate is an important part of life, but no particular relationship is a life or death proposition. "Let's be sensible," says the pragma lover.

MANIA is perhaps the least pleasant of the love styles to experience. A typical manic lover hungers for love yet expects it to be painful. There is no preferred physical type and, indeed, a manic lover may react negatively to someone at first meeting and then turn right around and become obsessed with that person. There is a lot of daydreaming about possibilities with a partner; much of a manic relationship is played out in the head of the manic person. There is a wish to see the partner constantly, great anxiety over what the partner might be doing (or who the partner might be with) when not with the manic person, and a feeling of loss of control and impending doom whenever the two are apart. Sometimes, if no particular problems exist, the manic lover seems to manufacture problems, pushing for more commitment or for further declarations of love and devotion and never seeming to feel really loved for more than a moment at a time. Loss of sleep, threats of suicide, and frantic phone calls are all signals that a partner is a manic lover.

AGAPE, the last and the rarest of the love styles, comes from the religious tradition of self-sacrifice for the welfare of others. It might be called "gift" love, for it takes no thought of the self but instead focuses on what is good for the partner. It accepts and values the partner simply for being in the world. Agapic love is more spiritual than physical. Although sexuality is not denied, it is not central to this love style; in any case, an agapic partner would be more concerned with the partner's sexual pleasure than with his or her own pleasure. Agape truly is altruistic, and in this sense has a different focus from any of the other love styles. Whereas ludus and pragma seem rather focused on the self, and eros and storge are focused on the relationship or interaction, agape is focused on the partner. Given the lofty requirements of agapic love, it is not surprising that Lee found no pure agapic types in his research. (These descriptions of the six love styles have been adapted from Hendrick & Hendrick, 1992a, pp. 99–101.)

Love Attitudes Scale

Based on Lee's (1973) theory and on some preliminary scaling work (Lasswell & Lobsenz, 1980), a measurement scale called the Love Attitudes Scale was developed to assess Lee's six major love styles (Hendrick & Hendrick, 1986). The complete scale is shown in Box 2.1. The scale contains 42 items, with seven items for each of the six love styles. Each set of seven items is averaged to yield a score for the particular love style. Thus, every person completing the scale achieves a score on each of the six styles. For discussion purposes, it is even possible to take the three most strongly endorsed subscales and construct a three-point "profile" for an individual.

B O X 2.1
The Love Attitudes Scale

Listed below are several statements that reflect different attitudes about love. For each statement, fill in the response on the answer sheet that indicates how much you agree or disagree with that statement. The items refer to a specific love relationship; answer the questions with your current partner in mind. For each statement:

>   5 = Strongly disagree with the statement
>   4 = Moderately disagree with the statement
>   3 = Neutral, neither agree nor disagree
>   2 = Moderately agree with the statement
>   1 = Strongly agree with the statement

Eros
1. My partner and I were attracted to each other immediately after we first met.
2. My partner and I have the right physical "chemistry" between us.
3. Our lovemaking is very intense and satisfying.
4. I feel that my partner and I were meant for each other.
5. My partner and I became emotionally involved rather quickly.
6. My partner and I really understand each other.
7. My partner fits my ideal standards of physical beauty/handsomeness.

Ludus
8. I try to keep my partner a little uncertain about my commitment to him/her.

9. I believe that what my partner doesn't know about me won't hurt him/her.
10. I have sometimes had to keep my partner from finding out about other partners.
11. I could get over my affair with my partner pretty easily and quickly.
12. My partner would get upset if he/she knew of some of the things I've done with other people.
13. When my partner gets too dependent on me, I want to back off a little.
14. I enjoy playing the "game of love" with my partner and a number of other partners.

Storge

15. It is hard for me to say exactly when our friendship turned into love.
16. To be genuine, our love first required *caring* for a while.
17. I expect to always be friends with my partner.
18. Our love is the best kind because it grew out of a long friendship.
19. Our friendship merged gradually into love over time.
20. Our love is really a deep frienship, not a mysterious, mystical emotion.
21. Our love relationship is the most satisfying because it developed from a good friendship.

Pragma

22. I considered what my partner was going to become in life before I committed myself to him/her.
23. I tried to plan my life carefully before choosing my partner.
24. In choosing my partner, I believed it was best to love someone with a similar background.
25. A main consideration in choosing my partner was how he/she would reflect on my family.
26. An important factor in choosing my partner was whether or not he/she would be a good parent.
27. One consideration in choosing my partner was how he/she would reflect on my career.
28. Before getting very involved with my partner, I tried to figure out how compatible his/her hereditary background would be with mine in case we ever had children.

Mania

29. When things aren't right with my partner and me, my stomach gets upset.

30. If my partner and I break up, I would get so depressed that I would even think of suicide.
31. Sometimes I get so excited about being in love with my partner that I can't sleep.
32. When my partner doesn't pay attention to me, I feel sick all over.
33. Since I've been in love with my partner, I've had trouble concentrating on anything else.
34. I cannot relax if I suspect that my partner is with someone else.
35. If my partner ignores me for a while, I sometimes do stupid things to try to get his/her attention back.

Agape

36. I try to always help my partner through difficult times.
37. I would rather suffer myself than let my partner suffer.
38. I cannot be happy unless I place my partner's happiness before my own.
39. I am usually willing to sacrifice my own wishes to let my partner achieve his/hers.
40. Whatever I own is my partner's to use as he/she chooses.
41. When my partner gets angry with me, I still love him/her fully and unconditionally.
42. I would endure all things for the sake of my partner.

NOTE: Names of the love styles are shown for each group of items. In a research study, participants are not told that there are six love attitudes but are simply asked to fill out the scale.

The Love Attitudes Scale can be useful in couple counseling, but it should be used to "describe," not to "diagnose." There are no established norms for the scale that will indicate that certain profiles are linked with marital dissatisfaction, psychopathology, and so on. The scale can be administered, scored, and then used to tell partners how they are similar and dissimilar. To give a general idea about how people score on this measure, average subscale scores for married couples in one research study are shown in Table 2.1 (Contreras, Hendrick, & Hendrick, 1994). The couples in this study were divided into three groups based on cultural identification: Hispanic-oriented, bicultural, and Anglo. It is apparent that all three groups of couples had relatively similar scores on the subscales of the Love Attitudes Scale. Such findings should be of interest to therapists who work with couples of various cultures because the results indicate that love is experienced similarly in different cultures. People can be so much the same when it comes to love.

Extensive research has been conducted with the Love Attitudes Scale, but only selected findings most relevant to counseling couples will be

TABLE 2.1
Couple Scores on Love Attitudes

Subscale	Anglo couples	Bicultural couples	Hispanic-oriented couples
Eros	2.10	2.10	1.96
Ludus	4.22	3.74	3.72
Storge	2.13	2.29	2.43
Pragma	3.24	3.29	2.83
Mania	3.98	3.65	3.85
Agape	2.21	2.14	2.03

NOTE: N for ethnicity = 54 Hispanic-oriented subjects, 54 bicultural subjects, and 60 Anglo subjects. The lower the score, the greater the endorsement of the subscale

presented here. The experience of falling in love is somewhat different from that of loving in an ongoing relationship. In exploring whether people who reported themselves to be in love would differ in their love attitudes from people not currently in love, Hendrick and Hendrick (1988) found that people in love were higher on eros and agape and lower on ludus than were people not in love. Thus, those in love were more passionate and altruistic and less game-playing. The two groups also differed on several other measures. If a therapist were to administer the Love Attitudes Scale to a couple and find that one or both partners scored more strongly on game-playing than on either passion or altruism, the therapist might evaluate the couple differently than if both were very altruistic.

Women and men differ in how they approach many aspects of their close relationships. In fact, the theme of gender differences runs through this volume. The area of love is no exception. Over time, there have been a number of gender differences in love styles, though not all of them have been consistent. For the most part, women are more inclined to be friendship-oriented (storge) as well as practical (pragma) in their approach to love, and they are also somewhat more possessive and dependent (mania). Men, on the other hand, always appear more game-playing (ludus) than women. That does not mean that therapists should automatically look for gender differences in couples seeking treatment, but differences that do appear need to be acknowledged and dealt with.

Although men and women do differ in some respects in how they experience, men also differ from each other, just as women do. In fact, in one study (Bailey, Hendrick, & Hendrick, 1987), gender role, as measured by the Bem Sex Role Inventory (Bem, 1974), showed more scale differences than did actual gender, prompting the conclusion "that one's sex-role orientation or one's attitudes and values about the 'meaning' of male and female may be more important than whether one actually 'is' male or female, at least in regard to love attitudes" (Hendrick & Hendrick, 1992b, p. 71).

Some love research has attempted to look at individual personality-type characteristics that might be related to love style preferences. Self-esteem is one such characteristic, and the finding most relevant to counseling is that people who are higher in self-esteem are less possessive and dependent (mania) in their love attitudes and more passionate (eros) (Hendrick & Hendrick, 1986). This fits with the images of an intense but secure and confident eros lover as contrasted with the vulnerable, insecure mania lover (who is likely to appear in a therapist's office). Self-disclosure is also related to love. Research showed that passionate lovers were most disclosing to a love partner, and altruistic lovers were also disclosing. However, game-playing (ludus) lovers were the opposite (Hendrick & Hendrick, 1987). Ludus likes to maintain distance, and that is incompatible with any meaningful self-disclosure. Thus, if a couple in counseling took the Love Attitudes Scale, and one or both partners was endorsing of ludus, it is likely that rather guarded communication (and minimal self-disclosure) would be characteristic of that relationship. What ludic partners might score highly on, however, is sensation seeking. A ludic partner gets bored easily and requires a lot of excitement and novelty in a relationship (Hendrick & Hendrick, 1987; Richardson, Medvin, & Hammock, 1988).

Although it is interesting to consider how personality is intertwined with attitudes toward love, a therapist is more likely to be concerned with what is already known about the love styles of couples in ongoing relationships.

Love in Continuing Relationships

Although only a little love styles research has been done with partners in relationships, the findings are interesting. A study of dating couples (Hendrick, Hendrick, & Adler, 1988) explored the love styles as predictors of relationship satisfaction and relationship adjustment. The strongest positive predictor of satisfaction and adjustment for both relationship partners was the passionate love of eros. In addition, game-playing was a negative predictor for men and possessive dependence a negative predictor for women. When couples who stayed together were compared to couples who broke up, the continuing couples were higher in passion and lower in game-playing than were the breakup couples. Similar results were found for a group of married couples (30 Anglo, 27 bicultural, 27 Hispanic-oriented) (Contreras et al., 1994). Across both genders and all three groups, passionate love was the strongest predictor of marital satisfaction.

Such results may seem surprising to those who expect that passionate love occurs only at the beginning of a relationship and inevitably disappears as the relationship continues through years of day-to-day living. "Often we equate length of marriage (or chronological age) with romantic intensity, e.g., young/newlywed = passionate; older/married longer = companionate. However, many middle-aged couples will be happy to report that love involves not so much 'getting older' as 'getting better,' and one of the things that may get better is passion" (Hendrick & Hendrick, 1992b, pp. 95–96).

Just as passion is not the exclusive property of the young, however, companionship and friendship are not the exclusive property of the mature. Recent research analyzing college students' written accounts or "stories" of their important love relationships (Hendrick & Hendrick, 1993) revealed some unanticipated findings. Based on three studies and 84 accounts, it appears that friendship (the storge love style) is the most frequently occurring theme in accounts of intimate relationships. In addition, when participants were asked to write about a close friendship, about half the time they wrote about their romantic partner. So the lines between passionate love and friendship love are blurry for young couples as well as older ones. Both types of love are essential to relationship initiation, development, maintenance, and success. Both couples and their therapists would do well to remember that passion and companionship are not mutually exclusive.

It is clear that many factors are involved in beginning and maintaining an intimate, partnered relationship. The following case example illustrates how problems can beset a relationship even when the relationship basics (for example, similarity, commitment) are all in place.

❧ *Case Example* ❧

Carol and Bob are a married couple who have recently begun couple counseling. Carol is 29 and a high school English teacher, while Bob is 31 and an accountant. They have been married for five years and have one child, a daughter, age 3. They entered counseling because of what they reported as a "growing distance" between them; they have long periods of relative quiet, punctuated by arguments. The arguments are typically initiated by Carol, who states that she is finding fewer and fewer rewards in the marriage. Both partners state that their sex life is satisfactory (though less so than in the past), that they love each other and their daughter, and that they want to try to recover what they have "lost" in their relationship.

Their first three counseling sessions have been spent in gathering individual and joint family histories, and they have filled out several questionnaires, including the Love Attitudes Scale. The following is their fourth counseling session. Text in brackets is related to theoretical and research material discussed earlier in the chapter.

Therapist: So, how are things going?

Carol: Well, I'm feeling a little better. We've been talking more this past week. I guess that when we talked about how we got together and what our courtship was like . . . well, we remembered why we fell in love in the first place.

[Carol had lost sight of some of the rewards in the relationship.]

Bob: I never forget why we got together, but still, it helps to remember all those early times. And to remember what our childhoods were like and how similar we are in some ways but how different we are in others. Carol's family . . . (Carol interrupts)

Carol: My family is very different from Bob's family. Oh, I know that the two families live in the same city and seem similar, but they are really very different. My family is warm and expressive; they make a big fuss over things like holidays and birthdays—they make everyone feel "special." Bob's family—well, they are just much more reserved. I never know quite where I stand with them.

[Partners have both similarities and differences.]

Bob: Carol, that's not true! And besides, your family is so emotional—they make a fuss over everything.

Carol: Yes, it is true. After all this time, I don't even know how your mother really feels about me.

Bob: What do you mean? She loves you like you were her daughter.

Carol: She never says that. Oh, I know she's always pleasant to me, and if we need help, she's always there, but . . . (she shrugs)

[Issues that were not important at one relationship stage become important at another stage.]

Therapist: Let's stop for a minute and look at what has been going on here. Carol, you have been feeling some emotional distance from Bob, and you talk about some of the same things in regard to his family. There's nothing specific you can point to—but you don't feel as close or as intimate as you'd like to. Bob, you're pretty bewildered about all this, and when Carol gets upset, you just want to soothe her so that things will calm down. But you try to talk her out of her feelings rather than find out why she might be feeling a certain way. Remember, both of you, last week you filled out the Love Attitudes Scale, and then I gave you some information to read about the love styles. Well, I have your results, and they fit right in with what we are talking about. Here, each of you look at your results for a few minutes.

[Gender differences: Women may want to talk about hurt feelings, but men may back off from conflict.]

Bob and Carol each look at their Love Attitudes Scales and scores, including the three-point code of their most-endorsed scales. Carol's code is E/S/P, meaning that eros (passionate love) is her strongest scale, followed by storge (friendship love), and then pragma (practical love). Bob is an S/A/E, meaning that storge is his strongest scale, followed by agape (giving love), and eros.

Therapist: What do you think?
Carol: When I went home last week, I read the information you gave us about the love types. I guess that from what little I know, these types here really fit for me. I am an eros—although I am also really concerned about friendship in marriage and also about practical things. But I think love should be exciting, not all the time, but sometimes. When we started dating, I thought Bob was handsome and sexy and romantic—and I still think he's handsome and sexy. I know that being married and having a child change things a lot, but romance doesn't have to just die—does it?
Therapist: Bob, how are you reacting to this?
Bob: I think these love styles fit pretty well. Carol really is more romantic than I am, I guess. What's most important to me in our relationship is our friendship; Carol and I have always been "best friends." But love and sex are important to me too. I miss some of the magic we had when we were first together. But mostly I just want to get back to being happy together.
Therapist: What you are each saying is consistent with these love style results. Romance and passion are important to both of you, but more so to Carol. Friendship and stability are also important to both of you, but more so to Bob. You really aren't that far apart when you talk *to*

rather than *at* each other. And it helps to understand the other person's intentions.

[Therapist uses love styles to help each partner reframe the other partner's behavior.]

Therapist: Carol, if Bob seems more interested in companionship than romance at times, you may tend to think, "I'm not attractive to him anymore" or "He doesn't love me as much as he used to." When really, he's just being a storgic lover who values friendship and companionship a lot. And Bob, if Carol sometimes seems to want more intensity than you do, you may tend to think, "She's unhappy with me" or even "She's just being overly emotional, like her family." And really, she just wants some romantic intimacy with you. There is no substitute for talking things out and asking the other person what they are feeling and thinking. But it is also useful to begin changing some of your behaviors. Tell me, when was your wedding anniversary?

Carol: It was last May. Why?

Therapist: Did you give each other presents? And if so, what?

Bob: I gave Carol a subscription to a magazine about food and health. We are both interested in that.

Carol: I had flowers sent to Bob at his office. But he told me later that he got a little embarrassed.

Therapist: It sounds like, Carol, you gave Bob a perfect eros gift and, Bob, you gave Carol a perfect storge gift. The problem is, you each gave the gift you really wanted to get. There's nothing so unusual about that, but I'd like you to try doing things a bit differently. I have some homework for you. I want you to pick a day next week to be your unanniversary day. I want you to decide together how you will spend the evening, and I want each of you to pick out a gift that is appropriate for the other person, based on their love styles. Then at our next session, I want you to come back and tell me how it went. How does that sound?

Bob: It sounds good to me.

Carol: Me too.

Therapist: Good. Then we'll meet again next week.

This dialogue is just a slice of a therapy session and compresses a lot of information into just a few interchanges. But it does show how different family characteristics and communication patterns as well as a difference in love styles (or relationship priorities) can influence a partner's perceptions of self, the partner, and the relationship. Even for a couple whose problems are much more serious than Bob and Carol's, love issues may well be core issues.

Summary

Finding a partner and constructing a relationship are not easy tasks. People typically choose partners who are similar to themselves, who have a number of desirable characteristics, and who will engage in a process of mutual exploration and disclosure to develop intimacy and trust. It is important for the relationship to be rewarding. This process is governed by individual partner characteristics, aspects of the dyadic interaction, and social network and societal influences. Love is a necessary requirement for the continuation of most romantic relationships. At one time it was thought that passionate love followed by companionate love was the predictable course of events for a long-term romantic relationship, but it may be that passionate loving and companionate loving are both important all during the life of a relationship. In addition to being passionate and companionate, love can also be described as game-playing, practical, obsessive, and giving.

CHAPTER THREE

Negotiating Intimate Relationships

Lisa and Phil had been dating for almost a year and had been sexually involved for about the last four months. They had become progressively more intimate, sharing their attitudes and values, cultivating the same friends, and generally intertwining their lives. Although they were physically attracted to each other and enjoyed the sexual aspects of their relationship, as they became emotionally close and even began to talk about a long-term commitment, they decided that sex made their feelings about each other less rather than more clear. So they decided to stop having intercourse (though other physical affection was okay), at least until they were more definite about their future.

Sexual Aspects of Relationships

Love and sexuality are two areas of a relationship that are at least moderately intertwined. Of course, it is possible to have love without sex, and "it is possible to have good sex, even excellent sex, without love. However, the *best* sex occurs within the context of love, which, in turn, will nearly always involve a relationship with another with both sexual and nonsexual aspects" (Hendrick & Hendrick, 1992a, p. 115). So it is particularly appropriate to consider sexuality within the context of a close relationship. Sex is one reason couples seek counseling; it may underlie or may actually be the presenting problem. In working with couples on issues of sexuality, it is useful to have a framework, or perhaps several frameworks, in which to place these issues.

Sex During Courtship

Sprecher and McKinney (1993) have noted three orientations toward sexuality that encompass most peoples' attitudes and values toward sex. These include procreational, relational, and recreational orientations. Those holding a procreational orientation believe that the purpose of sex is to create life—to reproduce. The relational orientation emphasizes sex as a means of expressing affection and increasing intimacy in a close relationship. The recreational orientation offers sex as an enjoyable activity without the need for "strings to be attached." This book embraces a relational orientation, because therapists working with couples are most likely to deal with sexual issues in the relational arena. Couples in which both partners agree that reproduction is the reason for sex are unlikely to seek counseling (an exception occurs with infertility), and couples in which partners take a recreational view of sex will probably not seek therapy (although one partner's recreational view is likely to bring a nonrecreational partner for help). In any case, it behooves a counselor to understand the partners' individual and joint orientations to sexuality early on in the counseling process.

Sexual attraction. Sexual attraction is a major component of romantic love, and physical attractiveness is an aspect of that component (Hatfield & Sprecher, 1986; Hendrick & Hendrick, 1992b). However, as noted earlier, beauty is typically in the eye of the beholder, so selective factors cause people to become attracted to some potential partners but not to others. And both physical and sexual attraction may be more important to some types of lovers. Remember, the passionate eros love style involves intense physical attraction and a strong desire for intimacy, whereas storge is oriented to friendship and stability. Research exploring love attitudes and sexual attitudes found that the eros love style was associated with an idealistic and communication-oriented approach to sexuality (or what might be thought of as a relational orientation), whereas game-playing ludus love was related to both a permissive and instrumental approach to sexuality (more like the recreational orientation) (Hendrick & Hendrick, 1987).

There also appear to be some gender differences in sexual attraction. Women and men may be in relative agreement about many of the qualities they find desirable in a partner, but in some research men ranked "physically attractive" more highly than did women, while women thought "good earning capacity" and "college graduate" were more important than men thought they were (Buss & Barnes, 1986).

Another predictor of sexual attraction is a partner's level of sexual experience, and that is linked to the sexual "double standard." The idea of a "double standard" refers to the belief that while it is permissible for men to have premarital sexual experience (especially intercourse), it is not permissible (or at least less permissible) for women to have such experience. There has been some conjecture that the double standard is fading, and indeed, some scholars have found women's and men's sexual mores to be converging (Curran, 1975). However, in a recent study, when people were asked to evaluate men and women of different ages who supposedly had intercourse in either a serious or a casual relationship, women were evaluated more negatively for having sex at a younger age or for having casual sex (Sprecher, McKinney, & Orbuch, 1987). Women are apparently still expected to be more sexually "selective" and to wait longer for sex, although it is clear that attitudes toward both premarital and extramarital experience for women and men continue to evolve.

Not only may a partner's sexual past become a point of contention in a current relationship, a partner's behavior in the present relationship may also create conflict. For example, if Phil and Lisa, mentioned at the beginning of the chapter, had sexual relations fairly early in their dating relationship and are now moving toward a commitment to marry, Phil could develop some nagging concerns about the fact that Lisa had sex with him so readily. These concerns may not be easily recognizable—even to Phil himself—but they may result in his provoking arguments, questioning Lisa's fidelity, and even being extremely jealous of her or devaluing her. Thus, qualities and behaviors that originally draw partners together become the very things that later divide them.

Some couples engage in sexual behavior that stops short of intercourse. Reasons for this may vary from religion or value standards to fear of pregnancy or sexually transmitted diseases. However, for those who do engage in intercourse, the "first time" is likely to be considered a turning point or significant event in a couple's relationship (Baxter & Bullis, 1986). A number of factors influence partners as they move toward this first time. Four general reasons to have sex were outlined by Christopher and Cate (1984) and include (1) positive affection/communication (love), (2) arousal/receptivity (being "turned on"), (3) obligation and pressure (one partner pressures the other), and (4) circumstantial (drinking too much). Although both partners may be motivated by these and other reasons to become sexually involved, typically women are somewhat more motivated by the affection/relationship-oriented reasons whereas men are more likely to respond to physical factors (Sprecher & McKinney, 1993). These gender differences in sexual motivation can usefully be kept in mind when courting (and married) couples are experiencing sexual conflict. Sexual events in the relationship may have had somewhat different meanings for the two partners, and these meanings may have changed for the partners themselves over the course of the relationship. (For example, sex may become an expression of intimacy for the male partner and a great tension release for the female partner whereas earlier in the relationship the reverse was true.)

Although most of the couple examples here have used heterosexual couples, gay and lesbian couples also experience many of these same sexual problems, as well as some issues more common to same-sex relationships. For example, men in our society tend to be socialized to more actively seek sexual involvement, while women have done less initiating. Thus, a gay male couple may feel that they need to over-initiate sexually (thus creating pressure), while lesbian partners may initiate less than is actually desired (Berzon, 1988). (For additional discussion of same-sex couples see Kurdek, 1992; Kurdek & Schmitt, 1986.)

There are various possible reasons for sexual conflict, and frequency (or rather infrequency) of sex is one that therapists hear relatively often. It is tempting at this point to refer to statistics on average frequency of intercourse for various types of couples and try to talk about what is "normal." What is likely to be of greatest interest to a counselor, however, is the meaning that such frequency has for relationship partners seeking help. What may have been viewed by a woman early in the relationship as her partner's "passionate nature" may have been negatively reframed (Dattilio & Padesky, 1990) as "he always wants sex." This becomes just one more nail in the relationship's coffin. Actual frequency rates vary widely, both within age groups and across age groups, in length of relationships, and so on. But much more relevant to a therapist is the relative satisfaction partners feel with intercourse frequency and with other aspects of their sex lives.

Satisfaction

If partners agree on the frequency with which they have intercourse—or even agree whether or not to have intercourse at all—this will not be a source of conflict. Research found that some groups of couples differed in the amount and timing of sexuality, however the groups did not differ in relationship satisfaction (Peplau, Rubin, & Hill, 1977). Although other research has found that sexual frequency and satisfaction are linked (for example, Blumstein & Schwartz, 1983), still other work found that giving affection was more important to marital satisfaction than was sexual interest (Huston & Vangelisti, 1991). Thus, it is likely that partners helped by a therapist to express more verbal and physical affection to each other will become more satisfied, whether their sexual activity changes or not.

Some of the research findings just presented are based on dating couples and some on married couples. Many relational dynamics are similar for dating and married couples. Various sexual behaviors are related to sexual satisfaction, which in turn is related to general relationship satisfaction. But the actual behaviors are less important than the way in which they are perceived and interpreted by the partners. Therapists can work with relationship partners to improve their sex life, but it is equally or more important to help them perceive partial successes as just that—partial sexual successes rather than partial failures.

Areas of Negotiation

The whole sexual process can be thought of as one long series of negotiations; however, particular topics are more thorny than others. Surprisingly, perhaps, birth control may still be an area for negotiation, when it is talked about at all. There are still many abortions and unwanted pregnancies in the United States, even though considerable technology exists to prevent conception. There are various theories about why women fail to use contraception (Rains, 1971; Reiss, Banwart, & Foreman, 1975). Adler and Hendrick (1991) proposed that failure to contracept is due both to intrapersonal characteristics such as sexual self-esteem and to interpersonal characteristics such as love and sex attitudes and the quality of the romantic relationship. Research findings indicated that self-esteem and sexual self-esteem (intrapersonal factors) as well as a passionate orientation to love (an interpersonal factor) were all related to positive contraceptive behavior (Adler & Hendrick, 1991). Not surprisingly, partners who feel good about themselves, including their sexuality, are more likely to communicate about sensitive topics like birth control. And partners who are more oriented to each other and to the relationship may be better contraceptors also. But scholars are a long way from developing a really comprehensive model of contraceptive behavior, in spite of the importance to romantic partners of making consensual decisions about birth control. It is useful for therapists to keep in mind, however, that as partners feel better about both themselves and their relationship through the course of therapy, they are more likely to improve their contraceptive planning.

The topic of sexually transmitted diseases, specifically AIDS, is also problematic for couples. Although many couples do discuss their own and the partner's previous sexual experience, many do not. As noted earlier, women may still be judged more severely than men for having premarital sexual experience, so disclosure of past behavior may not be in one's immediate self-interest. Even the current fear of AIDS does not compel disclosure. Sprecher (1991) found that in a sample of 100 dating couples only about half said that due to AIDS they were more likely to ask their current partner about her or his previous sexual relationships. Although people's reluctance to talk about sex may seem unusual, therapists are unlikely to be surprised by the difficulty many couples have in dealing with sexual negotiation, whether about problem areas or just about everyday aspects.

Married Couples

Although much of what is known about the sexuality of courting couples can also be applied to married partners, there are some differences. For one thing, frequency of intercourse typically declines during the course of a relationship, and these effects are likely to be felt primarily in married relationships. In fact, it has been estimated that rates of lovemaking decline by about one-half during the first year of marriage (James, 1981). That is the bad news. The good news is that it may take 20 years for such rates to halve again. And many couples actually enjoy sexual activity more in midlife (when childrearing responsibilities or the fear of pregnancy are no longer at issue). In fact, as discussed earlier, it was found that for both Mexican American and Anglo married couples, the strongest predictor of marital satisfaction was having a passionate orientation toward love (Contreras et al., 1994).

Sexual quality may not decrease over time, but sheer quantity of sexual activity does in fact decrease with length of marriage. One reason for this is that the novelty of sexuality, and even of the relationship itself, wears off. However, as therapists who work with couples know, novelty can be recreated. A change in the timing (morning instead of evening), location (living room instead of bedroom), and position (side-by-side instead of missionary) of intercourse and other sexual behaviors can re-create considerable novelty for an otherwise reasonably contented couple.

How sex feels is very important, but as we noted earlier, what it means is perhaps more important. Sex is just one element in a close relationship, and it can mean many things. It may be self-disclosure (being naked both emotionally and physically), a way of being intimate, a way of expressing love and affection, an expression of closeness and interdependence, an act of relationship maintenance (maintaining or nurturing the relationship), and an exchange behavior (doing something positive for each other) (Sprecher & McKinney, 1993). Thus, when counseling a couple with sexual problems, a therapist needs to determine the meaning of sexuality to each partner and help the partners communicate these meanings to each other. Communication itself can be the most important sexual behavior.

Sexuality is an important positive element in an intimate relationship. But it may also be a forum for relationship destructiveness.

Sexual Coercion

Sexual coercion is not confined to dating or to married or even to heterosexual relationships; it spans all romantic relationships. Sprecher and McKinney (1993) define sexual coercion broadly as sexual activity that may range from exploitation to aggression to assault and rape.

In dating couples, sexual coercion may occur at many levels. Christopher and Frandsen (1990) found that men were more likely than women to report employing pressure and manipulation strategies as sexual influence techniques in dating. Elsewhere it was found that men were more likely to perpetrate sexual abuse in a dating situation, whereas women were more likely to be the victims of sexual abuse (Burke, Stets, & Pirog-Good, 1988). Reasons for coercion include miscommunication between partners and assumptions about what certain behaviors mean. Part of this miscommunication is that women (and men) may sometimes say "no" to sex when they actually mean "yes" (Muehlenhard, 1988; Muehlenhard & Hollabaugh, 1988). Therefore, when a "no" is really a "no," it is not taken seriously by a partner, even though it should be.

Although there has been considerable research on date rape (for example, Koss, 1988; Shotland, 1989), a counselor working with couples may be more concerned with ongoing sexual coercion in a relationship than with a specific instance of sexual assault. Many states have no laws protecting a wife from unwanted intercourse with her husband, though more and more states are enacting such legislation. The dynamics of sexual coercion are similar to those of other types of physical abuse, and before any useful couple counseling can occur, the abuse—or sexual coercion—must cease.

One influence on sexual coercion is sexual miscommunication. This is the flip side of the positive communication that must occur if sex is to be really satisfying. No matter what facet of a close relationship is examined, communication always seems to be involved.

Communicating in Relationships

Every close relationship involves communication, both verbal and nonverbal. Sexuality in a relationship involves ongoing negotiation, but the relationship itself must also undergo continual negotiation and renegotiation if it is to survive and prosper. And negotiation involves communication. It is likely that in relationships where there is little communication there is also little negotiation. Relationship rules have been written in stone, and they do not change.

Types of Communication

People place tremendously high expectations on communication, often seeming to expect it to miraculously remediate all kinds of relationship problems (Fitzpatrick, 1988a). Even though limitations are placed on communication by relationship power, gender role attitudes, and so on (see

Chapter 5), communication is still expected to work wonders. Two kinds of communication are expecially important to intimate relationships: nonverbal communication and self-disclosure.

Nonverbal communication. "Body language" includes posture and body movements, facial expressions, eye contact, and the like. Behaviors such as eye contact can be used to accelerate intimacy but can also be used to dominate (Kleinke, 1986). It can be very useful in couple counseling to ask each partner to do an informal analysis of the other partner's nonverbal behaviors, pointing out characteristic behaviors and their inferred meaning for the partner doing the analysis. Some partners are surprisingly astute in "reading" their partner's nonverbals. And other partners are surprisingly dense. In either case, the exercise can be useful. Working with a married couple in which the husband would go off on tangents while the wife got progressively more bored, one day the therapist observed that the wife began filing her nails while her husband was talking. That behavior was more informative to the husband than the wife's previous verbal statements had been.

Self-disclosure. In the preceding chapter, self-disclosure was mentioned as a vehicle for promoting the development of a dating/courting relationship. It is also an integral part of an ongoing relationship. A recent review of the self-disclosure literature pointed out that both relationships and self-disclosure are subjective and dynamic and thus mutually transformative (Derlega, Metts, Petronio, & Margulis, 1993). Various relationship factors may influence disclosure, which may in turn influence these factors. How partners define their relationship (superficial versus intimate, stable versus unpredictable) may influence disclosure. For example, disclosure is likely to be deeper in a stable, intimate relationship than in an unpredictable, superficial one. Time or the length of the relationship also matters. Self-disclosure is typically seen to develop gradually over time (Altman & Taylor, 1973), although sometimes relationships "click" very quickly and disclosure develops rapidly (Berg & Clark, 1986).

The attributions or explanations that are constructed for various relationship behaviors also affect disclosures, as does one partner's affection for the other partner. For example, if someone cares deeply for a partner, that individual may be more likely to disclose positives but less likely to disclose negatives. Degree of reciprocity can also affect disclosure, and finally, the partners' goals for the relationship will likely influence the kind and amount of self-disclosure. For example, if further intimacy is desired, one or both partners is likely to disclose more. If one partner wants to keep his or her distance, disclosure is cut off.

Gender and Self-Disclosure

Perhaps one of the greatest influences on self-disclosure is gender. Decades of debate have addressed how similar or different women and men are in the area of disclosure (Derlega et al., 1993). Most findings indicate that women are more conversational and disclosing in same-sex friendships than are men, although men can be more disclosing when they are interacting with someone they might wish to date (Caldwell & Peplau, 1982; Derlega, Winstead, Wong, & Hunter, 1985).

Recently, scholars have introduced the intuitively appealing argument that women and men are essentially raised in different subcultures and that these subcultures have different agendas for communication (Derlega et al., 1993). It can be argued that different values are placed on disclosure in men's and women's subcultures, that there are different (and gender-related) social norms about appropriate disclosure for women and men, and that different things are expected "by" and "from" men and women concerning the behavior of self-disclosure.

Self-disclosure is more a part of women's lives than of men's lives all during development. For example, traditionally it has been acceptable for girl children to cry and then talk about their hurts, whereas boy children were told (either verbally or nonverbally) to be quiet and stoic. Because disclosure is more a part of girls' than of boys' development, it is seen as more appropriate for adult women than for adult men. Women are thus "allowed" to disclose about personal things, whereas men are not. And, indeed, research shows that the penalties are higher for men who break "appropriate" gender role norms than for women who do so (Seyfried & Hendrick, 1973). So men typically do not break the rules about disclosure; they tend to keep things inside. Not surprisingly, because disclosure is more a part of the fabric of women's than of men's lives, it may be valued more highly by women. Women expect it to accomplish more as a positive relationship behavior. Men are not as comfortable disclosing, don't do it as much, and are not as good at it. Men are not necessarily anti self-disclosure; disclosure may simply be unfamiliar or may just not be all that relevant.

Although these differences exist, it is important that the descriptions not be drawn too tightly. In fact, gender differences in self-disclosure are not particularly large, even though they may be fairly consistent (Dindia & Allen, 1992). Therapists have seen both the stereotypes—and their opposites—in action. It is not uncommon to interview relationship partners and to have the woman be much more willing to talk than is the man, although the reverse also occurs. Sometimes a woman may talk "at" a man, in which case there may not be a great incentive for him to respond. However, each partner can be taught specific communication skills (discussed later in this chapter) to improve both their verbal and nonverbal communication.

But it would be foolish not to recognize that men are impeded (sometimes by themselves, sometimes by the culture) from developing skills and comfort with the process of self-disclosure. Female partners, couple counselors, and men themselves can modify the sociocultural messages that restrict men from the relational and healthful (Pennebaker, 1990) benefits of self-disclosure, but such messages must be recognized before they can be changed. Therapists can be helpful in illuminating these messages during counseling, saying that although the culture may not support men's self-disclosure the therapist does.

In addition to gender differences in disclosure and communication, there are also couple differences. Fitzpatrick (1988b) has categorized couples on the basis of their interaction style. *Traditionals* are interdependent, share many things, and communicate nonassertively for the most part. *Independents* also do a great deal of sharing, but they have autonomous lives and may be quite assertive and even confrontive in their communication. *Separates* are much less interdependent than either of the other couple types, have limited assertiveness in their communication, and avoid open conflict. It is useful for a couple therapist to keep these couple types in mind. Although communication is important for a relationship, different types as well as different levels of communication are appropriate for different couples.

Communication and Satisfaction

Links have certainly been drawn between relationship satisfaction and self-disclosure. Both marital and general life satisfaction have been related to greater disclosure (Burke, Weir, & Harrison, 1976), and Hendrick (1981) found not only a positive relation between a couple's marital satisfaction and their self-disclosure but also between one spouse's disclosure and the partner's marital satisfaction. The higher one partner's disclosure, the higher the other's satisfaction. Still other research found that both disclosure given to a partner and perceived disclosure from a partner were positively correlated with marital satisfaction (Jorgensen & Gaudy, 1980). Although disclosure is not uniformly positive and too much disclosure about relationship negatives may increase dissatisfaction (Levinger & Senn, 1967), it is generally a relationship asset. Therapists typically will not go wrong if they help partners better express their thoughts and feelings, with a greater proportion of these positive than negative.

One problem in relationship communication is that one partner may be more accurate in hearing the negatives than in hearing the positives from a partner. Whether it is a comment about one's appearance or one's willingness to do a fair share of the housework, there is a tendency for positive comments to be noted and then discarded while negative comments are noted and noted and noted. In one research study, when partners attempted to reciprocate both negative and positive feelings that they thought their partners had previously expressed toward them, only the negatives were successfully reciprocated (Gaelick, Bodenhausen, & Wyer, 1985). And in similar research, Noller and Venardos (1986) conducted a laboratory study with couples reporting high, moderate, and low marital adjustment. When evaluating their ability to correctly interpret their partner's communications, high and moderate adjustment couples thought that sometimes they were accurate, sometimes not. And they were typically correct in knowing when they were on (or off) target. However, the low adjustment couples were confident about *all* the communications they interpreted, whether they were subsequently right or wrong. This inflexibility and self-confidence about being "right" was absolutely consistent with their lower adjustment. This is also consistent with what so often occurs in couple therapy—the unhappier the partners, the more each is convinced that he or she is "right."

Communication in a close relationship is a necessary but complicated venture. It sometimes seems like a tug-of-war. Baxter (1990) has discussed relationship development, including aspects of communication, from a dialectical perspective. In this perspective, competing, sometimes seemingly contradictory needs always exist in a relationship—needs that must be accommodated. Baxter cites three basic contradictions in relationships: autonomy-connection, openness-closedness, and predictability-novelty. The openness-closedness contradiction or dimension is most relevant here, for Baxter notes that relationships need information openness to facilitate intimacy yet need information closedness to constrain feelings of vulnerability. Although Baxter (1990) found that openness-closedness was a contradiction experienced more in initial stages of a relationship than in later stages, the relationships she examined averaged less than two years' duration. It is likely that the issue of openness-closedness may ebb and flow during the life cycle of a relationship, but in a vital relationship it is never completely static and probably never completely resolved.

Sexual Communication

Sexual communication can refer to how partners employ sexuality to communicate with one another, but here it refers specifically to communicating about sex. As noted earlier, it can be very awkward for partners to talk about sex.

Couples use words to initiate (or refuse) sexual interaction, though nonverbal methods for initiating sex are used even more frequently than are verbal methods (Brown & Auerback, 1981; Sprecher & McKinney, 1993). Research also indicates that men in intimate relationships are more often the initiators of sexual interactions, which puts women in the position of more frequently being the refusers. Of course, many times women initiate, and many times men refuse, but the predominant behaviors are predictably gender-stereotyped.

Couples may also use words to describe the sexual activities they are (or want to be) engaged in. Erotic words may be used to refer to sexual intercourse, other sexual behaviors, and parts of the body. Couples may develop their own "language" for sexuality, thus strengthening the unique aspects of the bond between the partners.

Research indicates that sexual communication satisfaction is linked to both sexual satisfaction and couple adjustment. After questioning more than 400 married individuals, it was concluded that sexual communication satisfaction influences sexual satisfaction, which in turn influences overall adjustment/satisfaction (Cupach & Comstock, 1990). Such conclusions are consistent with research discussed earlier linking relationship satisfaction to self-disclosure. It is not surprising that if general communication can contribute to relationship satisfaction sexual communication can be influential also.

Strategies for Better Communication

A detailed presentation of communication training for couples is beyond the scope of this book, but some basic therapeutic concepts and strategies may be useful. The material is consistent with both communications and cognitive-behavioral therapeutic orientations and has been drawn largely from Dattilio and Padesky (1990), Satir (1967), and Stuart (1980).

In beginning to work with a couple, the therapist needs to talk with the partners about how they view their communication. Do they think they have problems communicating? If so, when do these problems arise? What topics are problematic? When they are communicating the best, what is it like? What is it like when they are communicating the worst? Although a therapist might believe that almost complete openness between partners is the ideal, that level of communication might not work for some couples.

Although no single level of communication is right for all couples, clear communication is probably a viable goal for everyone. Partners communicate both verbally and nonverbally, but it is best to put things into words so that they can be understood accurately. Nonverbal behavior is subject to a great deal of misinterpretation, and when there is conflict between verbal and nonverbal channels of communication, the nonverbal channel is the more powerful (Stuart, 1980).

Stuart proposes four basic "rules" for effective couple communication. These include (1) listening attentively (being attentive, being patient, and letting the partner finish), (2) making requests constructively (using "I" statements, being direct but also polite), (3) giving selective and focused feedback (not saying every negative thing that comes to mind, timing the feedback effectively), and (4) being willing to clarify one's own messages and seek clarification of the partner's messages.

These skills can be effectively taught in a fairly standard couple communication exercise in which partners engage in discussion of an issue and take turns as speaker and listener (Dattilio & Padesky, 1990). The therapist serves as the "coach" during the interchange, stopping the discussion to correct, clarify, and offer suggestions. Partners can keep repeating a given exchange until they "get it right," with the therapist there to mediate. A variant on this exercise was suggested by Satir (1967) and has been modified slightly:

> Have relationship partners sit with their chairs back to back. Ask them to discuss a current issue in their relationship. After they have talked for a few minutes, have them turn around and face each other, making eye contact. Then ask them to discuss the same issue. Finally, ask them to hold hands and discuss the issue. Later, talk with them about the different ways of communicating, the back-to-back situation being much like what goes on at home, with one person making a negative comment as the other person is leaving the room, and the other two situations offering more constructive settings for communicating.

Many such exercises can help partners improve their communication, and therapy time spent in communication training is time well spent. To quickly assess how much partners are communicating/disclosing to each other, the brief communication scale shown in Box 3.1 can be employed.

BOX 3.1
The Self-Disclosure Index

Self-Disclosure to a Relationship Partner
With your current partner in mind, indicate how much you have disclosed to that person about the topics listed below. For each statement:

> 5 = Strongly disagree (have not discussed at all)
> 4 = Disagree
> 3 = Neutral
> 2 = Agree
> 1 = Strongly agree (have discussed fully)

1. My personal habits.
2. Things I have done that I feel guilty about.

3. Things I wouldn't do in public.
4. My deepest feelings.
5. What I like and dislike about myself.
6. What is important to me in life.
7. What makes me the person I am.
8. My worst fears.
9. Things I have done that I am proud of.
10. My close relationships with other people.

You can obtain an overall self-disclosure score by adding up the scores across the ten items. The lower the score, the more likely you are to have disclosed to your romantic partner.

NOTE: This self-disclosure questionnaire was developed by L. C. Miller, J. H. Berg, and R. L. Archer (1983). Openers: Individuals who elicit intimate self-disclosure. *Journal of Personality and Social Psychology, 44*, 1234–1244. Used by permission of Lynn Miller and the American Psychological Association.

This measure should be used descriptively in counseling, similar to the use of the Love Attitudes Scale discussed in Chapter 2. It may be useful for partners to know how similar they are in their levels of disclosure. To compare a particular couple's disclosure with that of other couples, average self-disclosure scores for participants in one research study are shown in Table 3.1 (Hendrick & Hendrick, 1988).

This chapter has explored in considerable detail the topics of sexuality and communication using as examples both dating and married couples. However, it is important to also recognize a group of couples increasing in both numbers and importance—cohabiting couples.

Cohabiting Couples

Cohabitation involves partners living together in a close relationship without being legally married. This arrangement appears to allow a certain amount of intimacy and stability while also allowing considerable partner autonomy, and indeed it is the modal relationship for couples who are gay or lesbian, who typically cannot legalize their relationships. Critics of cohabitation view it as a threat to the marital establishment. But Reiss and Lee (1988) point out that cohabitation is part of courtship and partner selection, not an alternative to eventual marriage. Although cohabitation may be an increasingly popular option for young couples who want to be together but who for one reason or another do not wish to marry, a number of studies have shown

TABLE 3.1
Self-Disclosure Scores for Women and Men

Measure	Women	Men
Self-disclosure to a lover	1.66	1.86
Self-disclosure to a friend	1.74	2.28

NOTE: N = 98 women and 106 men. The lower the score, the greater the endorsement of the scale.

that cohabitants may be somewhat less able to achieve marital success than noncohabitants (see DeMaris & Rao, 1992; Newcomb, 1986; Thomson & Colella, 1992).

A number of reasons have been proposed to explain why cohabitation does not lead to greater marital success, including the possibility that people who cohabit are less conventional and thus more willing to get divorced down the line or that the findings are really an artifact based on the greater time that cohabitants have been together. In any case, cohabitation is not a way of avoiding later marital failure; neither does it necessarily lead to such failure. The therapist dealing with partners who are living together should be aware that cohabitation has different meanings for different couples. For one couple it may represent a signpost on the road to eventual marriage. For another couple, cohabitation may itself be the end of the road. Sexual relating, communication, and all the other issues that affect dating and married couples are equally likely to occur when partners are cohabiting. So in many ways, cohabiting partners can be counseled just as any other couple.

But there are additional complexities. Cohabiting partners have less "institutional" commitment to each other than do partners who have entered into the institution of marriage. Levinger (1979) talked about barriers to relationship dissolution, and legal marriage is one such barrier. Couples who are cohabiting have one less barrier to breaking up. On the other hand, cohabiting partners may be much more involved in each other's lives (and possessions) than are dating partners. Indeed, some research indicates that cohabiting couples may have sex more frequently than do dating couples (Sprecher & McKinney, 1993). Thus, cohabiting couples have many characteristics in common with both dating and married couples yet occupy their own special place in the world of close relationships.

Sexuality is an important component of a close, romantic relationship, and negotiation of the sexual aspects of being together can be both exciting and awkward. Such negotiation can be aided by the partners' abilities to communicate with each other. However, failure to communicate, both sexually and nonsexually, is a common problem propelling couples into counseling. The following case example illustrates some of the issues discussed in this chapter.

ஃ *Case Example* ஃ

Daniel and Elena have been in a close romantic relationship for about three years, with most of that time spent living together. Daniel is 25 and a draftsman; Elena is a 24-year-old registered nurse. They entered counseling because of what they reported as a problem with "intimacy" in their relationship. It turns out that intimacy is by and large a synonym for sex, and sex (specifically intercourse) has become less frequent and less satisfying for both partners in the past couple of months. It is their dissatisfaction with the level of sexual and emotional intimacy in their relationship that finally brought them to therapy. They have expressed a wish to solve their sexual problems so that they can perhaps begin to talk about making a more permanent commitment. Their first four counseling sessions have been spent in gathering histories and discussing their sexual problems, which seem to focus largely on Daniel doing less initiating of sex because Elena seems less responsive. Each blames the partner for "causing" the downturn in their sex life. The following dialogue is from their fifth counseling session.

Therapist: How have things been this past week?

Daniel: Okay, I guess. Since you told us that at the beginning of counseling it is better to just be aware of behaviors rather than try to change them, I have felt less pressure about sex this week. But nothing has really changed.

[Pressure is a real contra-indication for good sex.]

Therapist: What did you hope would change?

Daniel: Well, I just thought that since we are trying to get help with our problems that . . . well . . . that Elena might be a little more interested in our being intimate.

Elena: What did you think was going to change? Did you think that just because we are seeing a counselor I would be ready to jump into bed whenever you're in the mood? There's a lot more to sex than that.

[Gender differences: Women may respond more to relational factors in sexuality, men to physical factors.]

Therapist: Elena, it sounds like you're afraid that Daniel won't take this whole situation seriously enough—that he will think everything's fine when you don't feel that way at all.

Elena: That's right! Whenever there's a problem, Daniel thinks that if we talk about it once for five minutes, then everything's settled. That's not enough.

Daniel: But, Elena, you want to talk all the time. (Turning to the therapist) She seems to think that talking will solve the problem.

[Gender differences: Women may want to talk more about feelings than men do.]

Therapist: Let's wait a minute. We started by dealing with you trying to lessen the sexual pressure and begin tracking what pleases each of you. Now we're talking about "talking." What do you think this is about?

Elena: (Sits quietly but nods affirmatively)

Daniel: What do you mean?

Therapist: I mean that you two may be experiencing some dissatisfaction with your sexual relationship, but I think that what's going on is as much about communication as it is about sex. Daniel, you are a can-do guy, and you are very competent and like to get to the bottom of things and not waste time. And talking about things can sometimes feel like a waste of time when you want to just get on with it. Elena, you are also a competent person who knows how to get to the bottom line, certainly in your work as a nurse, but you are also very person-oriented. You want to interact and talk about things, whether it's your relationship with Daniel or even just what the two of you each did at work during the day.

[Gender differences in self-disclosure again.]

Elena: Yes, I don't want to just sit around and talk all the time, but I do want to talk more than Daniel does. And that really bothers me. It happens with sex too. I mean, Daniel is great in bed—he's a wonderful, thoughtful lover. But he never says "I love you" or "I want to make love with you" or anything like that. He just puts his arms around me and kisses me and one thing leads to another. . . .

Daniel: But you know how I feel. Why do I have to endlessly tell you?

Elena: Not endlessly, just sometimes.

Therapist: Okay, I think you've got something. It seems that if no communication is a 0 and constant communication is a 10, Daniel is about a 3 or 4 and Elena is about a 7. Is that about right?

Daniel: Well, actually I'm more of a 5, I think.

Elena: I think so too. And 7 is about right for me.

Therapist: Okay, so we're not talking too far apart here. There are some differences, but they are not drastic. And they're perfectly consistent with what women and men in our culture do. Women are brought up to talk, to self-disclose. Men are brought up not to talk, at least not about really personal things. So men don't talk, women try to get them to talk, men back off, women pursue, and so on. Whichever way you look at it, it doesn't work to do it that way.

[Therapist highlights cultural messages about how men and women are supposed to communicate.]

Daniel: That's right. My Dad talks a lot about business and sports, but he never talks about his feelings. I would talk with my mother some when I was growing up, but only sometimes, not all the time. And one of the things that has always been special about Elena for me is that I have always been able to talk with her about anything.

Elena: (Looks surprised) I had no idea that you felt that way. I know that we have been able to talk about some things, but I never knew that our talking was so important to you. Sometimes when I try to talk to you, you seem to just shut me out. It's like a wall coming down, and I can't get through to you.

Daniel: I know what you're talking about. Sometimes you seem to want to talk about something longer than I want to, or longer than I can. Sometimes I get tired of talking and just want to get on with things. But other times things get so intense that I get scared.

Therapist: And when you get scared?

Daniel: When I get scared, then I need to spend some time by myself to think about things and regroup.

Elena: I know he needs that. And when I feel scared, I want to talk about it. So we are different that way.

Therapist: You are different that way. But you are also much alike. Neither of you is at an extreme, either extremely quiet or extremely talky. It seems to me that you have meshed pretty well for much of the time you have been together. But a few months ago you two started talking about making a permanent commitment, getting married. Maybe, Daniel, you got a little nervous, so you backed off to have time to think and regroup. And, Elena, maybe you got a little nervous too and wanted to talk about it. But your ways of coping with the nervousness really conflicted.

[Cohabiting couples have their own unique stresses.]

Daniel: I think that's true. And when I'd try to reconnect with Elena, usually by wanting to make love, then . . . (Elena interrupts)

Elena: Then I'd feel distance between us because we hadn't been talking as much to each other, so I wouldn't feel very romantic toward Daniel. Or when I did feel romantic, I would also feel angry.

Therapist: It seems like you two had a system going. You were really close to each other, so you talked about getting married. You each felt a little nervous at considering such a big life change, so you reacted in predictable and familiar ways, Daniel by withdrawing and Elena by wanting more. Then Daniel would reach out sexually, and Elena would be unavailable. You began to see the problems as sexual, but they are really much more about talking—and agreeing not to talk. You see, whether you talk or not, if you agree to it, you are still both in sync.

[Perceptions of a problem can be more of a problem than the problem itself.]

Daniel: And we're still both talking. I didn't realize that I could talk about not talking, like I could say "I don't want to keep talking about this right now." And maybe that would be okay with Elena.

Elena: Yes, most of the time that would be okay with me. I don't always have to continue talking about something if we aren't getting anywhere or it isn't working. I just want to be able to come back to it sometime later and try to resolve it then.

Therapist: All right. You two have done a lot of work today. This is a very important understanding that you have come to. You two can learn to communicate about your communication, sort of making rules about the rules. That way, when you aren't communicating well, you can talk about what is going on and change things—or stop for a while. That's enough work for today. We'll work more on communication during our next session.

[Partners can be taught improved communication skills.]

Clients in the "real world" seldom come to an understanding of communication so swiftly. These clients had only begun to communicate and had many more sessions, working on communication skills and also dealing with their individual and joint fears about intimacy and commitment. What happened in this session, however, put the focus of therapy squarely on the processes that were disrupting the relationship. And it was particularly useful for the partners to not only understand what was going on but to initiate new behaviors (in this case talking about talking) right in the therapy session.

Summary

Sexuality is intertwined with love in an ongoing romantic relationship. Sexual attraction means different things to different people. A passionate lover would feel strong sexual attraction to the partner, whereas a more friendship-oriented lover would value sex as just one of many relevant factors in a relationship. Although some scholars have predicted the demise of the sexual double standard, it appears that women are still judged more harshly than are men for having certain kinds of sexual experiences.

The first time that partners have sexual intercourse is likely to be a significant event in their relationship. Sexual satisfaction is linked to relationship satisfaction in some complex ways, and many areas of sexuality may be problematic (for example, STDs, sexual coercion).

Communication is central to relationships in our culture. Both nonverbal and verbal communication are important, and women tend to be more self-disclosing than men. Communication has been linked to relationship satisfaction. Sexual communication satisfaction may have an impact on sexual satisfaction, which in turn influences relationship satisfaction.

CHAPTER FOUR

Staying Satisfied

Lesha and Jerome had been married for 15 years. They had two children (ages 10 and 12) and were involved in a number of family-related activities. Although they considered themselves to be "best friends" as well as spouses, they worried that something might be missing from their relationship. Sometimes they felt that the "spark" was gone. So they saw a therapist. After working with them for several weeks and offering them various ideas for revitalizing their relationship, the therapist commented that the basic structure of their relationship seemed solid. Jerome and Lesha expressed satisfaction with their relationship, for the most part and found these comments reassuring. They said that they were glad to realize that it was not only acceptable for a relationship to look different at year 15 from the way it looked at year one—it was positively healthy.

 è.

Initiating and developing a relationship is extremely important, but it is equally important to focus on maintaining that relationship—what helps and what hurts. Although there is no clear line between relationship development and relationship maintenance, the latter refers more to factors that emerge in importance once a relationship has been launched and is ongoing. Many factors influence relationship maintenance, including those discussed earlier—love, sexuality, and communication. The focus in this chapter is on factors that may not appear in traditional texts on marriage counseling but which may be quite influential in strengthening or weakening relationship bonds. These factors include relationship satisfaction, conflict and negative attributions, and social support and friendship.

Relationship Satisfaction

Much has been written about marital satisfaction, though there is still some dispute among scholars about definitions of satisfaction. Is satisfaction the important concept, or is adjustment? Or quality? Which concept is meant, and how is it measured? These arguments may not seem critical to the therapist working with couples on the "front lines," however, a few distinctions are worth noting.

Different Terms, Different Concepts

As Glenn (1990) observed in a review of this topic, some scholars view the issue as "marital quality," which can be defined as married persons' subjective feelings about their marriage. These subjective feelings can, in turn, be referred to as the "satisfaction" perspective. On the other hand, marital quality has also been viewed as consisting of actual behaviors or characteristics of the marriage (for example, conflict or communication). This perspective can be thought of as the "adjustment" point of view.

From the practitioner's vantage point, it is probably wise to take a both-and rather than an either-or stance, depending on whether the therapist is interested in a couple's adjustment or their satisfaction. If a therapist wants to know how generally content people are in their relationship (beyond what is learned from therapy sessions), he or she might administer a brief satisfaction measure such as Hendrick's (1988) Relationship Assessment Scale (RAS), shown in Box 4.1. However, if a more comprehensive measure is needed, Spanier's (1976) Dyadic Adjustment Scale (DAS) is widely used. Interestingly, this 31-item measure correlates highly with the briefer RAS, demonstrating the difficulty of trying to differentiate satisfaction from adjustment—at least with a written measure. Other measures give a more fine-grained assessment of how a couple is doing (Snyder's [1979] Marital Satisfaction Inventory consists of nearly 300 items), but for most situations, briefer measures meet a therapist's needs.

The RAS can be used in couple counseling, but it does not have established norms that differentiate satisfied from dissatisfied couples. However, in one research study (Contreras et al., 1994), married couples who were Hispanic-oriented had a total score of 29.76, those who were bicultural scored 28.83, and Anglo couples scored 29.75. None of these couples were identified as dissatisfied, and all were very similar to each other in relationship satisfaction.

Beyond the theoretical issues and the measurement considerations, there is another important point to consider regarding the satisfaction/adjustment question. Assuming that a therapist is seeing a couple in therapy, is she or he interested in how the couple "feels"? If so, then satisfaction is what is needed. Or is the therapist more interested in what the couple "does"? In that case, adjustment may need to be measured.

Debating terminology is not strictly an academic exercise. The very words of description used for certain feelings or events influence the ways

---

B O X 4.1
The Relationship Assessment Scale

Please mark on the answer sheet the letter for each item that best answers that item for you:

1. How well does your partner meet your needs?

A	B	C	D	E
Poorly		Average		Extremely well

2. In general, how satisfied are you with your relationship?

A	B	C	D	E
Unsatisfied		Average		Extremely satisfied

3. How good is your relationship compared to most?

A	B	C	D	E
Poor		Average		Excellent

4. How often do you wish you hadn't gotten in this relationship?

A	B	C	D	E
Never		Average		Very often

5. To what extent has your relationship met your original expectations?

A	B	C	D	E
Hardly at all		Average		Completely

6. How much do you love your partner?

A	B	C	D	E
Not much		Average		Very much

7. How many problems are there in your relationship?

A	B	C	D	E
Very few		Average		Very many

NOTE: To derive a numerical score, A = 1 and E = 5. The greater the total score, the more satisfied. Items 4 and 7 are reverse-scored.

in which those feelings or events are thought about. For example, the word "adjustment" may be more value-laden and more negative than the word "satisfaction," and a therapist may find it easier to describe a couple as "less satisfied" rather than as "less adjusted." Some may disagree. Hopefully, therapists can learn more about couples' attitudes as well as their relationship behaviors without getting lost in the terms used to describe them.

Satisfaction Over Time

The issue of whether marital satisfaction or contentment exhibits predictable changes during the marital and family developmental cycle has been somewhat controversial. Much research indicates that satisfaction present at the beginning of a marriage decreases during the period of child-rearing, and then increases again during the empty nest stage (Rollins & Cannon, 1974; Weishaus & Field, 1988). This is referred to as *curvilinearity*.

One explanation for marital satisfaction being up, then down, then up again is the concept of "role strain" (see Burr, 1973; Rollins & Cannon, 1974). This concept refers to the stress people experience as they try to perform various (often multiple, sometimes disparate) roles. Role stresses result from both family and work obligations, both of which may be greatest during the middle, child-rearing years of marriage. Thus, there are logical explanations for a curvilinear relationship between marital satisfaction and length of marriage.

Partner Differences in Satisfaction

Another area of interest to therapists is the way partners may differ in satisfaction levels. When trying to determine how partners feel about their relationship, certain things become apparent right away. First, and not surprisingly, partners may differ in how satisfied or dissatisfied they are. One partner may be getting more from the relationship and feel relatively content, whereas the other partner, who is getting less from the relationship, is unhappy. Sometimes both partners are equally unhappy. In any case, individual differences exist in level of satisfaction.

What is more subtle and equally important to know is that there can also be gender differences in satisfaction. Sociologist Jesse Bernard (1972) described men's and women's differential experiences of marriage as "his" and "her" marriages. In some early research, married partners rated each other's behaviors for a two-week period on two dimensions: affective/instrumental (emotional/task-type) and pleasurable/displeasurable. Results revealed both gender similarities and gender differences. Wives and husbands reacted to displeasurable emotional and task behaviors in a similar fashion. However, when it came to pleasurable behaviors, men and women differed: husbands rated wives' task behaviors as more important, and wives rated husbands' emotional behaviors as more important (Wills, Weiss, & Patterson, 1974). For example, Anna and Julio are a married couple. Julio especially values the things that Anna does for him, like making his lunch or buying him a new CD. Anna, on the other hand, is most pleased when Julio really listens to her and supports her emotionally. These gender differences are rather ironic. Traditional gender roles have typically required men to exhibit more instrumental behaviors and women more emotional ones, yet women appear to want emotional behaviors from men who, in turn, want instrumental behaviors from women. Each wants from the other what is hardest to get!

Other selected research shows some gender differences in satisfaction. A study of love styles in dating couples (discussed in Chapter 2) found that for women passionate love and an absence of possessive or game-playing love predicted satisfaction. For men, passionate love, self-esteem, and an absence of game-playing love were the significant predictors of satisfaction (Hendrick et al., 1988). It seems that men and women share many similarities in relationship satisfaction, but similar does not mean "the same."

It is interesting to consider how satisfaction might work in same-sex couples. Considerable differences exist in the contexts in which homosexual versus heterosexual relationships are conducted. Society makes it tougher to maintain gay and lesbian relationships (Berzon, 1988). However, some research indicates that there are fundamental similarities between homosexual and heterosexual couples. For example, Kurdek and Schmitt (1986) found that gay male, lesbian, and heterosexual couples were similar in love for partner, liking for partner, and relationship satisfaction— three very important bases for relationship continuation and success. And other relationship research found that gay men and heterosexual men had similar love and sexual attitudes (Adler, Hendrick, & Hendrick, 1987).

A final question in regard to relationship satisfaction is "Why is it considered so important?" First, it is important in its own right. People's feelings about aspects of their lives are significant; feelings influence the quality of life as well as the behaviors that compose much of the ongoing fabric of life. Second, satisfaction/adjustment/quality is important because of what it may indicate about eventual relationship continuation or termination. Satisfaction can be an effective predictor of whether or not a relationship will survive (Hendrick et al., 1988).

There is no simple, one-way relationship between satisfaction and relationship variables. In fact, recent research found a reciprocal relationship between satisfaction and aspects of marital interaction; each influenced the other (Zuo, 1992). And satisfaction is not a perfect predictor; all therapists know couples who are unhappy but who stay together nevertheless.

However, therapists who make the effort to assess partner satisfaction and adjustment will be able to make more than an educated guess about the couple's future. Such assessment provides information about how partners feel (satisfaction). If they are reasonably satisfied, the therapist may employ brief therapy. If they are extremely dissatisfied, then longer-term therapy as well as more frequent sessions may be indicated. Assessment also reveals what partners do (adjustment). If they spend little time together, they may need to plan "dates" to see each other more. If they have a lot of conflict, they need to be taught to fight fair. Satisfaction may be difficult to define, but it is clearly important.

A Perspective on Conflict

Conflict can strongly influence success or failure in a relationship. There are many definitions of conflict. According to Brickman (1974), conflict exists in situations where people must divide up resources in such a way that the more one person gets the less another person gets. A more interpersonal definition proposes that conflict occurs when one person's actions interfere with another person's actions (Peterson, 1983). In close relationships, when two people live together, one person is always interfering with another. Conflict occurs in a variety of situations, and several different topics of conflict may occur during a single episode of ongoing conflict.

For example, a conflict that starts over a particular issue (Alicia gets home from work late, and her partner Carlos is upset) may transform into a conflict about power and control (Alicia accuses Carlos of trying to control her life), which in turn transforms into a conflict about commitment (Carlos says that if Alicia spends so much time at work and so little time at home, she must not be committed to the relationship).

In analyzing the stages of conflict, Peterson (1983) described a beginning stage (conflict is cued by particular events and may be responded to either by avoidance or engagement/involvement), a middle stage (where either negotiation or escalation can occur), and a conflict termination stage, which can produce any of the following options:

- *separation* (both partners withdraw)
- *domination* (one person "wins")
- *compromise* (each person gives in a little)
- *integrative agreement* (a creative solution is found that meets both partners' needs)

- *structural improvement* (major changes are made in the relationship that aid conflict resolution over the long term)

Although the basis for conflict may be fairly clear (that is, a conflict of interest on a behavioral or emotional level), the content of a given conflict situation can range from money to sex to in-laws to children to jobs. Behind any particular conflict situation there is often a larger issue such as power and control, commitment, or self-esteem. And behind the larger issue lurks basic concerns of attachment versus loss, trust versus insecurity, and so on.

Couples may react to conflict differently; arguing means different things to different people. Researchers studied both stable and unstable couples and found that even among the stable couples, some couples had high positives and negatives (conflict) and were designated *volatiles*, others had moderate positives and negatives and were called *validators*, and still others, with low positives and negatives, were labeled *avoiders* (Babcock, Waltz, Jacobson, & Gottman, 1993).

Couples may experience conflict for situational reasons (for example, a partner's unemployment) or because one or both partners uses fighting as a typical mode of problem solving (often because the partner's parents did much the same thing). Any therapist who works with couples is familiar with relationship conflict; it is often the reason a couple enters therapy. Books about conflict—what it is and how to handle it—are typically part of the therapist's armamentarium. In addition, conflict that escalates into physical abuse is much more openly dealt with than it was a few decades ago (see Gelles & Cornell, 1985; Straus & Gelles, 1990).

However, once situational crises, chronic fighting because of family-of-origin learning, or actual emotional and physical abuse have been accounted for, many couples still experience "guerilla fighting" rather than full-scale war in their relationships. Partners may come to a therapist because they are not getting along or because they are unhappy or even depressed, but they do not always identify conflict as the source of the problem. One or both partners spends a lot of time trying to figure out why the other partner behaves as he or she does, often assuming negative motivations for behaviors. One marker characteristic of such couples is their tendency to "assume" or "mind-read" when it comes to partner behaviors. Once a therapist has talked with such a couple for a while, it becomes clear that the couple is experiencing a lot of conflict (perhaps at a fairly low but chronic level) and that the conflict is tying up a lot of the relationship's energy. It may be that the partners need to learn to check things out with each other rather than try to read each other's minds. In this case, communication training (see Chapter 3) is the next step in therapy. However, there is an intermediate step to consider first. That step involves dealing with partner attributions.

Attributions and Conflict

A causal attribution "is an inference about why an event occurred or about a person's dispositions or other psychological states" (Weary, Stanley, & Harvey, 1989, p. 3). Attributions are made for one's own behavior as well as for others' behaviors and involve perceiving and then making inferences about those perceptions.

For example, Alicia is late getting home from work; Carlos perceives that she is late and makes the inference that other things are more important to her than getting home on time. Carlos feels both threatened and irritated, and when Alicia finally gets home, he criticizes her for being late. Alicia perceives only Carlos's irritation (not his emotional vulnerability) and makes the inference that he is trying to control her behavior. She believes that her reasons for staying at work are fully legitimate (and, in fact, couldn't be helped), but instead of explaining these reasons to Carlos (which she sees as giving in to his control attempts), Alicia reacts to his criticism by in turn criticizing him. He then perceives her as uncaring and makes the inference that she values her job more than she does their relationship. He snaps at her, she snaps back at him, and conflict is off and running.

Attribution involves making judgments about people and events and trying to assign causes for things; at bottom, it is about trying to make sense of the world. And it is that sense-making process that makes attribution so relevant to therapy (where sense-making is essentially the basis for all that goes on). No matter what the therapist's theoretical orientation and whether the attributions are described as cognitions or as transference, attributions permeate therapy.

A couple of other aspects of attribution are also important. First, positive attributions as well as negative attributions may be made about another person's traits or behaviors. Second, when making attributions about another person's behavior, there is a tendency to over-attribute the behavior to dispositional causes or things internal to the person (Carlos saying "Alicia is an uncaring person") rather than to the situation (Carlos saying "Alicia just got caught in traffic"). Such tendencies in making attributions should be kept in mind as we examine what we know about attributions by partners in close relationships.

The Importance of Attribution

Much of the conflict in close relationships occurs when partners have different perceptions about each other's behavior and what causes it. Extensive research with couples indicates that the ways in which partners judge each other's behaviors is influenced both by whether the behavior is positive or negative and by the partners' satisfaction with the relationship. When dating partners evaluated themselves and each other, they said that their own negative behaviors were due to transient, situational causes but that their partner's negative behaviors were due to basic attitudes or personality characteristics (Orvis, Kelley, & Butler, 1976).

For married couples, unhappy partners were more likely to minimize or dismiss a partner's positive behaviors while exaggerating the partner's negative behaviors. The situation is quite different for more satisfied, non-distressed partners who were more likely to attribute a partner's positive behaviors to enduring internal factors (Jacobson, McDonald, Follette, & Berley, 1985). One problem with negative attributions is that they translate into less supportive and less effective relationship behaviors, which may increase the spiral of negativity in the relationship (Bradbury & Fincham, 1992).

Implications for Therapy

Based on the various findings concerning attribution-making by couples in close relationships, therapists have drawn some conclusions regarding the implications for therapy. When dealing in therapy with relationship partners who appear to be experiencing chronic (often low-level) conflict and who spend considerable energy making assumptions (often negative) about why the partner does certain things, some attribution work may be called for.

First, it is important to identify the specific relationship behaviors that distress one or both partners and that lead to conflict. Next, the therapist needs to help partners "check out" with each other the intentions of these behaviors as well as the ways in which the behaviors were interpreted. This is all part of the communication skills training discussed in Chapter 3. These steps of identifying the conflict-producing sequence and then clarifying intentions (that is, what Carlos meant to say) as well as perceptions and inferences (that is, what Alicia heard and the subsequent conclusions she drew) takes time and patience. It could be very useful during this process to explain the concept of attribution and the process that all people go through in trying to make sense of their own and significant others' behavior. Couples need to understand that it is normal to make attributions, but if this proceeds without periodic clarification, the process can get relationship partners in trouble.

Overall, in working with couples, it is important to remember the variables (for example, self-disclosure) that contribute positively to relation-ship satisfaction as well as the relationship conflicts that inevitably arise. Partners' abilities to be supportive to one another as well as their ability to just "be friends" can contribute much to relationship success.

Social Support and Friendship

The phrase *social support* has been popularized within the close relation-ships literature only in the last decade or so. Early work focused on suppor-tive social contacts and how these might contribute to personal adjustment (Cobb, 1976) and even serve as a buffer against various disease processes. Social support is no one thing but includes size and density of one's social network, availability and responsiveness of individuals within the network, and an individual's ability to make use of the network's resources (Derlega et al., 1991). Wortman and Dunkel-Schetter (1987) proposed the following list of important social support behaviors:

- expression of positive emotion toward someone
- support of someone's feelings and beliefs
- encouraging someone to express feelings
- offering information or advice to someone
- providing material aid to someone
- aiding someone with particular tasks
- helping someone feel a part of a group of people who will support each other

From this list, it is apparent that social support may be offered in emotional, cognitive, or behavioral terms.

In considering social support, it is extremely important to assess not only the support that may be available to an individual but also how sup-ported that individual actually feels. The term *perceived social support* has been used to refer to "the belief that if the need arose, at least one person in the individual's circle of family, friends, and associates would be available to serve one or more specific functions" (Cutrona, Suhr, & MacFarlane, 1990, p. 31). The importance of perceived social support should never be under-estimated. Most therapists have probably had clients in situations in which the knowledge that they had a safety net (perhaps consisting of only one person) was enough to keep them balanced on their particular tightrope. The net may not have had to be used—but the client had to know that it was there. Sometimes that net is the therapist.

Social support has been measured in a variety of ways, including having research participants fill out questionnaires, list persons in their social networks, or participate in a structured interview. Recent research has pointed out that social support is best considered as two constructs rather than one, with one construct encompassing perceptions of general support available to the individual and the other construct focused on the availability of support in particular intimate relationships (Pierce, Sarason, & Sarason, 1991). General perceptions of available social support may be a part of more stable frameworks or schemas with which people view their world, while relationship-specific perceptions of support may be more dependent on actual interactions with a particular relationship partner (for example, partner, parent, friend). Alicia may perceive that she has a lot of social support from her family and friends (general support) but may feel unsupported by Carlos (relationship-specific support).

Social Support in Intimate Relationships

Recent research explored social support in 50 married couples (Cutrona & Suhr, 1994). The couples were assessed on marital adjustment (using Spanier's [1976] DAS), social support, depression, and selected personality characteristics. Partners were also asked to interact in a social support task and after the task to evaluate each other in terms of supportive behaviors during the task. The authors were interested in social support communication behaviors in a number of areas, however those most relevant here are the ways in which individuals evaluated their partner's attempts at providing support.

Women tended to base their rating of their husband's supportiveness on his social support behaviors during the social support task. Neither women's marital adjustment nor the husband's supportiveness "generally" were important in the current ratings. For husbands, the reverse was true. "Among men, regardless of the number of support behaviors they received from their wives, their ratings of interaction supportiveness reflected their level of marital satisfaction and perceptions of their wife's supportiveness before the interaction began" (p. 22). Thus, for husbands, it didn't matter if wives were "perfect" during the interaction; only the outside behavior mattered. And for wives, it didn't matter if husbands were perfect "outside"; only the interaction behavior mattered. An additional finding was that emotional support was generally more appreciated than was informational support (advice) by both wives and husbands.

It may be natural for people to impose some constraints on the kinds of support desired as well as the timing of such support, but those who offer support may not always understand these constraints. Relationship partners may insist on being "helpful," whether the help is desired or not. Sometimes social support simply doesn't work, largely due to miscommunication or misattribution. And just as someone may not experience a behavior as supportive because it is not the right behavior at the right time, so also he or she may simply not "see" a supportive behavior.

Research with college students and their mothers found that students who had generally positive expectations of their mother's supportiveness were more likely to evaluate current behavior as supportive, whereas students experiencing conflict with their mothers perceived current supportive behavior as less supportive (Pierce, Sarason, & Sarason, 1992). So behavior may not be viewed as supportive if it comes into a nonsupportive context, and partners involved in couple therapy may have to be reminded frequently about each other's supportive behaviors.

Social support is complex. It is not as simple as one relationship partner just helping the other. Different types of social support are appropriate at different times, and the existence of support is no more important than the perception that the support exists. In addition, women may need to generalize from specific instances of male partner support, and men may need to focus more on specific instances of female partner support. Particularly relevant to therapy is that support may not be valued as highly if it comes into a context that is conflictual and nonsupportive. It is clear that negative attributions may be made about positive supportive behaviors unless the meaning of those behaviors (both intended meaning and received meaning) is made clear between relationship partners. Given that emotional support is virtually always evaluated positively, fostering emotional support is probably a good starting place for a therapist who is helping relationship partners learn to behave more supportively to one another.

Partners as Friends

Although close relationship researchers have studied extensively how adult friendships are formed and maintained, there has been less focus on the friendship aspects of intimate romantic relationships. In his review of the close relationships literature on friendship, Sherrod (1989) noted that while men and women seem to want the same qualities in a close friend (acceptance, trust, intimacy, and help), they may define these qualities in somewhat different ways and may also undertake the process of friendship somewhat differently. For instance, both women and men may seek social support and stress reduction in their friendships; they merely seek them by different means. Considerable research shows that men's friendships are much more concerned with activities, whereas women's friendships are more communication-oriented.

Such differences are likely to have an impact on intimate romantic relationships in which partners are friends as well as lovers. In heterosexual couples, women may want to engage in more intimate conversations, while men want to be active and "do things." These tendencies are likely to be accentuated in gay male or lesbian couples, wherein the former may be especially action-oriented and the latter especially talk-focused (Berzon, 1988). Such tendencies are not necessarily a problem, but understanding them can help relationship partners maintain better balance. (For an extended review of adult friendships, see Blieszner and Adams, 1992.)

Whether this topic has been studied formally or not, relationship partners are often close friends, if not best friends. As discussed in Chapter 2, research analyzing college students' written accounts of their love relationships found that a friendship-based orientation to love was the dominant theme expressed (Hendrick & Hendrick, 1993). In addition, when writing about a close friendship, nearly half the participants wrote about their romantic partner. There is a common phrase about "friends becoming lovers" and "lovers becoming friends," but in everyday human relationships, one's lover and one's friend are likely to be the same person.

Many variables are involved in maintaining a satisfying relationship, including consistent communication, construction of positive attributions, active provision of social support, and recognition that friendship may be an important part of the relationship. The following case example highlights some of these issues.

❧ *Case Example* ❧

Kathy and Joan have been in an intimate romantic relationship for the past seven years. They met in college, and began living together while in graduate school. Kathy is 28 years old and has a masters of social work degree. Joan is a 29-year-old attorney. They describe their relationship as beginning with a strong friendship and then growing into a deeper, romantic relationship. Both women are open about being lesbian and have good relationships with family members and most coworkers. They have come to counseling because their relationship, especially their communication, has deteriorated drastically over the past six months. They have always served as each other's "best friend"; however, they now live in silence most of the time. Kathy has been away from home, ostensibly at the office, and Joan believes that Kathy is going to leave her. Joan initiated therapy to try to maintain the relationship. Kathy protests that she does not want to leave the relationship, though she agrees that things cannot continue as they are. Each woman is quite expressive in talking to the therapist but "shuts down" when talking to her partner. They are in their second session.

Therapist: So, it appears that you both are expressing some strong wishes that the relationship continue, even though you are each unhappy with the way things are now.

Joan: Yes, I want us to stay together. But I just don't think that Kathy really does. Otherwise, she wouldn't behave the way she does toward me.

Kathy: (Sits quietly, but therapist notices that her fists are clenched)

Therapist: Kathy, how are you feeling right now? I notice that although you are not saying anything, your fists are clenched.

[Therapist comments on nonverbal behavior.]

Kathy: I get so angry when Joan doesn't listen to what I say because she thinks she knows better. I have just given up trying to talk to her, and sometimes I think that we will not be able to work this out . . . even though I want to.

Therapist: I understand that you are frustrated, but, Kathy, I am going to ask you to try talking just one more time. If you could be guaranteed that Joan would listen to you and really understand what you are trying to say, what would you say to her?

Kathy: (Kathy turns to Joan, who is quiet and appears to be listening intently) I do not want to leave—I really don't. But I get so frustrated with you and our relationship that I sometimes don't know what I'm going to do. You don't listen to me; you never have. Just because you have the prestige job and make more money than I do, just because you are supposed to be the "thinking" one in the relationship and I am supposed to be the "feeling" one, you assume that you are always right and that you always know better.

[Kathy has made attributions about Joan's power in the relationship.]

Joan: You say that you just don't know what you're going to do. What does that mean? (Joan begins to look more tense)

Kathy: You never listen to me. (Kathy looks angry)

Therapist: Wait a minute. I know that what you two are talking about is important, but something equally important just happened here. Kathy, I heard you express several things to Joan: one, you value the relationship; two, you get frustrated with things; and three, you believe that Joan doesn't listen to you or take you seriously a lot of the time. Is all that reasonably accurate?

[Therapist works on communication skills.]

Kathy: Yes.

Therapist: Joan, what you seemed to hear was only number two, that Kathy gets frustrated. You didn't hear number one or number three. Right away you started looking more tense and worried.

Joan: Yes, that's true. When I hear anything about her being frustrated or unhappy, I start thinking right away that she is getting ready to leave. And I don't hear much else.

[Joan makes negative attributions.]

Therapist: This is a key pattern in your relationship, I think. Kathy, you try to tell Joan how you are feeling. Joan, you hear only the negatives. You believe that Kathy is "really" saying that she wants out of the relationship, and you don't hear any more. Kathy, you then feel unheard and undervalued and attribute this to a power difference in the relationship, with Joan having more power than you do. So you, Kathy, shut down, and then you, Joan, become absolutely convinced that Kathy doesn't love you anymore. So then Joan pushes for contact, whereupon Kathy tries to tell Joan how she is feeling, and the cycle continues. Am I getting close to some of what is going on?

[Dissatisfied couples focus on the negative, so the therapist clarifies things.]

Kathy: Yes, this is part of what happens. I have real frustrations about the relationship, and I want some things to change. I'm not the shy college girl that I was when I met Joan. I am a successful and confident woman, at least a good part of the time. In fact, although I haven't told Joan about this, one of the reasons I've been spending so much time at work lately is that I am probably going to get promoted, so I simply have a lot of extra work to do.

Joan: I had no idea that you are getting promoted; that's wonderful! (Turning to the therapist) You are right about my not being able to really hear Kathy, at least not for a while. I get so stressed when she closes me out that I am not very rational about things. I certainly do not feel in control of myself, much less of our relationship. (Turning to Kathy) I can't believe that you think I have more power in our relationship. I don't feel that way at all.

Kathy: Some things have to change, but I don't want to leave you.

Therapist: Joan, what do you hear Kathy saying?

Joan: (Turning to Kathy) I hear you saying that we have some problems but that you want us to work things out. That is what I want too.

Therapist: Okay. Let's stop here. You two have started the process of talking with each other instead of at each other, but it is going to take a while. You need to do some work on your communication, but first it is important to understand that you have been doing a lot of attribution-making with each other. To try to explain a behavior, we can either ask someone why they are doing something, or we can make attributions or assumptions about it. Often our assumptions are negative—like Joan assuming that Kathy was staying at the office because she wanted to avoid being at home. If we are unhappy in our relationship, we are more likely to pay attention to negative events and almost ignore positive events. That is what has been happening with the two of you. Ideally, relationship partners check things out with each other instead of making assumptions, but once communication gets cut off, attributions, especially negative ones, can get more and more extreme. You have a number of issues to talk about and work on, but you took the first step today by really listening to each other for the first time in a while.

As with other fictionalized case examples, this looks too neat and tidy. However, this situation has some characteristics that make early conceptualization and intervention possible. For one thing, the relationship partners are both committed to making the relationship work. They may not be able to hear each other say that, but the therapist can hear it. For another, Kathy and Joan enact one of their dysfunctional communication sequences during the session, and the therapist is able to observe, stop, comment on, and reshape the sequence. Although these educated clients are particularly amenable to attribution work, nearly everyone can work with the idea of "checking things out" with their partner versus trying to "read their partner's mind." The language level may change, but the meaning is the same.

Summary

Whether it is defined as relationship satisfaction or relationship adjustment, the healthiness and successfulness of relationships is a major concern to couple therapists. It appears that marital satisfaction dips during the middle, child-rearing years. Men and women may be the same in terms of their levels of satisfaction with a relationship, but they may differ in the characteristics that influence that level. Conflicts exist in virtually all intimate relationships, and there are various ways to deal with them, including avoiding them or trying to communicate about them. Even if partners avoid talking about problematic events, they are likely to think about the events and make attributions about why the events occurred and why the partner acted in a certain way. And whether couples are satisfied or dissatisfied strongly influences the types of attributions made. This tendency to try to make sense of events is very normal, but partners who do not check out their attributions and assumptions with each other are likely to have serious problems at some point.

Partners who are satisfied with each other are likely to be friends as well as lovers and to provide each other with various kinds of psychological and physical social support. Such evidences of caring are very important in close relationships.

CHAPTER FIVE

Changing Rules and Changing Relationships

Dorothy and Roger are in their mid-forties. They have been married for more than 20 years and have two teenage children. They consider themselves a "contemporary" couple, and they share most of the decision making for their family. However, many of their activities fit into stereotypical gender-based categories. For example, Dorothy does most of the cooking; Roger mows the lawn. Some of Dorothy's friends tell her that by doing all of the cooking, she's really not the feminist she claims to be. Dorothy disagrees—but sometimes she wonders if they are right.

ॐ

This example could have included the endless combinations of activities that occur with couples today. Roger could have been described as sexist because he doesn't cook or as a wimp because he does. Or Dorothy might have been described as a "radical" feminist if she does all or most of the yard work. The fact is, many partners in relationships today feel "damned if they do and damned if they don't," seeming always to do either too much or too little, at least in the eyes of society.

Everywhere people turn, whether to television and movies or to the print media, they are deluged with messages about what they "ought" to do or think or feel. Sometimes they wonder if the world, and the intimate relationships in it, has changed too much—or too little.

Part of what troubles couples today is that relationship rules and norms have changed dramatically and continue to change (see Goldberg, 1985). Many of the changes date from the women's movement of the 1960s and 1970s, though the seeds of social change were planted much longer ago than three or four decades. Although the changes have been intended to improve the lot of women, such changes can be threatening to both women and men alike.

This evolving perspective on men and women is symbolized by current social science usage of the word "gender" in situations where "sex" would have been used formerly. The word *sex* is understood to mean biological sex, or the physical reality of having been born female or male. The word *gender*, on the other hand, "refers not only to biological sex, but also to the psychological, social, and cultural features and characteristics strongly associated with the biological categories of female and male" (Gilbert, 1993, p. 11). If we focus on sex, we are typically confronted immediately with unchangeable realities (for example, he is taller and heavier, she can bear children). Gender, on the other hand, permits analysis of the myriad interactions and interconnections of the fact of biological sex and all the characteristics and assumed characteristics that go with it (see also Deaux, 1993; Gentile, 1993).

Perspectives on Gender

Some current viewpoints on gender are especially useful for therapists. Gilbert (1993) outlines three ways in which gender can provide a lens through which to view the world. First, she describes the "gender as difference" approach that focused on the differences between women and men, whether in visuo-spatial ability, aggression, or leadership. The bulk of the difference findings (when any were found at all) seemed to favor men. However, a subsequent backlash occurred, and while some scholars seek to minimize gender differences, other scholars (for example, Belenky, Clinchy, Goldberger, & Tarule, 1986; Gilligan, 1982) seek to explain what differences there are by almost glorifying women. However, glorification of "women's" ways of doing things is really just the flip side of glorification of "men's" ways of doing things, and both keep the notion of "gender as difference" alive (Tavris, 1992).

Whatever the direction of thought on gender differences, it has always been easier to publish results that show "difference" rather than results that show "no difference." Thus, substantial bias exists in the social science literature toward research that shows gender differences. This is one area where the consumer had best beware. To magnify such differences is as unrealistic as to deny that they exist at all. Thus, "gender as difference" should probably be viewed with considerable wariness.

Gilbert (1993) also talks about "gender as structure," meaning that gender is an organizing framework for the distribution of authority, power, position, and economic resources. American society (as most societies) is patriarchal. When viewed through the gender lens, it is no surprise that men hold more power and resources than do women. What may be a surprise, however, is that gender continues to subtly influence many if not all assumptions about the social structure. For example, social and organizational sexism is responsible for much of the career inequity between men and women (Hendrick & Hendrick, 1992a). Gilbert (1993) notes that "employed men with children are still viewed as men, but employed women with children are considered mothers" (p. 15). Such an attitude is evident in the foreword of a marital therapy book (Goldberg, 1985) that talks about mothers making the choice to stay at home with young children or to work outside. What about fathers? Do they make choices?

The third perspective on gender is that of "gender as interactive process" (Gilbert, 1993) and refers to the ways in which thoughts about gender feed back to influence behaviors, which in turn modify thought patterns. To use the example that opened this chapter, if Dorothy believes that men are entitled to be taken care of, including being cooked for, then she feels responsibility to cook for Roger without expecting Roger to reciprocate. She may then feel burdened when she cooks, but guilty when she doesn't. On the other hand, if she feels that she and Roger need to each do a fair share to keep the marriage/family going, she may do the same behavior (cook) but may feel less burdened. She may also negotiate with Roger to share cooking and other chores. Recent research reported that mothers' stereotypic beliefs about gender influenced their perceptions of their male and female children's abilities (Jacobs & Eccles, 1992). The same might have held true for fathers; unfortunately, only mothers were included in the sample.

Gender influences thinking and behaving in myriad ways and cannot be ignored as therapists work with couples. Therapists' own personal lifestyles are bound to affect the ways in which they look through the gender lens. Are they married? Are they cohabiting? Is their relationship homosexual or heterosexual? Are they traditional or egalitarian? Because the answers to these questions have implications for how a therapist approaches couple counseling, it is important that therapists not fail to take gender into account in their work with couples, or in their own lives for that matter. (For more on gender, see Walters, Carter, Papp, & Silverstein, 1988.)

Power Issues

It is impossible to discuss the topic of gender without also examining the issue of power; the two are intertwined. Most social science presentations of the construct of power refer to the classic work of French and Raven (1968) that outlined five bases of social power:

- reward (one person can reward another)
- coercive (one person can punish another)
- legitimate (it is perceived as "appropriate" that one person has power)
- referent (one person has power by being likable)
- expert (one person has special knowledge)

Looking at the image of the traditional family in which the man is the sole breadwinner, it is not surprising that men had most types of power. Only in terms of referent power did women have the edge. As noted earlier, family structures are changing along with changing gender roles, and in fact, some would argue that the stereotyped traditional family was never a reality for the majority of families (Scanzoni et al., 1989). However, none would argue with the proposition that men have had and continue to have more power to gain and distribute resources than women have. Such a statement is not meant as an end point for discussion but rather as a starting point for therapists working with couples. When couples are seen in therapy, it is important to be aware that power is typically not equally shared between relationship partners.

Formerly, research on marital power was concerned with the resources that each partner brought to the relationship or which partner talked more during a decision-making discussion. But more recently the focus has been on the power strategies that women and men use with each other. Research with heterosexual and homosexual couples showed that although homosexual women and men did not differ significantly in their use of power strategies, heterosexual women and men did differ, with men reporting more direct and negotiating strategies and women more indirect and nonnegotiating ones (Falbo & Peplau, 1980). It was proposed that because women do not expect to have much power in influencing their male partners, they do not even bother to try negotiating strategies.

Howard, Blumstein, and Schwartz (1986) examined power strategies in a somewhat different way, identifying six power strategies or tactics that they divided into: weak power tactics (supplication, manipulation), strong tactics (bullying, being autocratic), and neutral tactics (bargaining, disengagement). They found that the clearest difference in use of power tactics occurred for weak tactics and depended on the sex of the person receiving the influence. In other words, "men elicit perceived manipulation and supplication from both female and male partners. The power associated with being male thus appears to be expressed in behavior that elicits weak strategies from one's partner" (p. 107). Although women and men have traditionally exerted power in somewhat different ways, changing gender roles inevitably imply changes in power.

Changes in Power

Sagrestano (1992) examined men's and women's power strategy choices under various experimental conditions. Participants were matched with a hypothetical partner (a female or male) and either (a) both partners had equivalent knowledge about the situation at hand, (b) the participant was an "expert," or (c) the participant was a "novice." Although Sagrestano expected that men would choose more direct and negotiating strategies while women would choose more indirect and nonnegotiating ones, that did not happen. There were *no* gender differences. The five strategies selected most by both men and women were persuasion, reasoning, discussing, asking, and persistence—four of which are direct and negotiating. There indeed were differences in choices of strategies, but these were made on the basis of amount of power that the participant felt he or she had. More and more research is showing that when women and men feel that they have equal power in a situation, they will use similar power strategies (Steil & Weltman, 1992).

Implications for Therapy

These findings have immediate implications for couple therapy. Lena and Jesse, a couple in their thirties, come in for therapy. One of their presenting problems is that Lena doesn't feel respected by Jesse (she doesn't feel she has an equal say in things), and Jesse frequently feels sexually rejected by Lena (when he initiates sex, about half the time she refuses). This problem could be framed as "He doesn't listen to her, so she retaliates by refusing to have sex with him" and handled as a communication issue. But it works just as well to frame it in terms of power. Based on what is known about power, it is possible that Jesse has more types of social power (for example, reward, coercive, legitimate, and expert) in the relationship and that Lena exerts referent power through emotional means. Thus, on many different issues, Jesse assumes that he "knows it all," and Lena, though resentful of this, wields the only power she feels she has—emotional/sexual power.

The way this couple communicates about issues is also interesting. Jesse, as the self-styled expert, tends to do a lot of telling and even a little bullying. Lena tends to plead and cajole, sometimes manipulate, and sometimes go off and do what she wants to do without consulting Jesse at all, leading him to feel excluded. This example may seem a bit stereotyped or even out of date, but it is still representative of many couples.

Since it is becoming more apparent that women and men who have equal power will use similar power strategies and will be more likely to negotiate directly with a partner, a therapist working with Jesse and Lena may try to "level the playing field of power," at least in therapy. Helping both partners acknowledge their current ways of getting power as well as their dissatisfaction with the results, then empowering Lena to be more direct with Jesse and working with Jesse to get his esteem needs met by something besides dominating Lena are reasonable therapeutic strategies. Having the partners "change places" and role-play a current conflict in their relationship might highlight the process. Whatever the therapist chooses to do, the key idea is to be aware of power imbalances (especially subtle ones) that sabotage relationships.

Although the topic of relationship violence was addressed briefly in Chapter 1, the focus there was on assessment of violence and needs for referral or reporting violence to authorities. Here, relationship violence is linked to both power and gender roles.

Power and Violence

Explanations for spouse abuse can be loosely grouped into personality-related factors, stressors, and social norms (Gelles & Cornell, 1985). Personality-related factors may include alcohol and drugs, mental illness, feeling threatened by change (including changes in gender roles or in power distribution), and difficulties with sex, communication, self-image, and so on. Stressors such as unemployment, poverty, and limited education can also accelerate abuse though, in fact, abuse crosses all ethnic, racial, and socioeconomic lines. The third area, social norms, is really the most related to power. Men's violence toward women, just as men's power over women, has been institutionalized in many cultures (Gelles & Cornell, 1985). Institutional acceptance of intimate violence is no longer so widespread in this culture. And some research indicates lower intimate violence rates in 1985 than in 1975 in the United States (Straus & Gelles, 1990). But changing gender roles and increasing power for women do not guarantee a lessening of violence.

Babcock, Waltz, Jacobson, and Gottman (1993) examined power and violence in marital relationships among three groups of couples: domestically violent, maritally distressed/nonviolent, and maritally happy/nonviolent. They compared various facets of power represented by economic resources, decision-making power, communication patterns, and communication skill. Husbands who battered their wives engaged more in a husband demand/wife withdraw type of interpersonal interaction than did other husbands. This is the reverse of the typical sex-stereotyped pattern that occurs during couple conflicts (that is, wife demands/husband withdraws). In addition, "poor husband communication, as well as discrepancies in education and decision-making power favoring the wife, were also associated with husband-to-wife aggression" (p. 47). It appears that an abusive relationship is more likely (all things being equal) where both partners have poor communication skills and the husband feels one-down in terms of power. Other research on the influence strategies of battered wives points out that battered wives are not necessarily passive (Frieze & McHugh, 1992). In fact, women who were married to violent men used a lot of influence strategies. However, the strategies were largely reactive and defensive ones. And the husbands who used violence as a power strategy also made the most decisions and held the most power.

So where does that leave women? If women are at greater risk for abuse when men have the power but also at greater risk for abuse when they themselves are perceived to have the power, then the only reasonably safe arrangement seems to be when both women and men have relatively equal power. Therapists who are sensitive to these issues can avoid reinforcing stereotypic power imbalances in couple therapy.

Power is also linked with date rape, another form of intimate violence. Although a detailed discussion of sexual abuse and even courtship violence is beyond the scope of this book, it is important to remember that men are more likely than women to use certain power strategies in the sexual arena. In one research study, men, more than women, were likely to have used manipulation and pressure to try to get a partner to engage in sex on a recent date (Christopher & Frandsen, 1990). And reports that occasionally make the evening news describing the gang rape of a college student by members of a Greek organization seldom report a man being sexually abused at a sorority party. The perpetration of a sexual crime is typically done "to women by men" and is about power just as surely as it is about violence.

If a couple comes in for premarital counseling, and the issue of sexual coercion is raised (he pressures her into having sex when she does not want to), the issue can be conceptualized as one of sex, or communication, or power—or all three. The issue may indeed be one of different desired frequencies for sexual activity, or the partners may simply not feel comfortable in talking about sex with one another. Just as likely, however, sex is the field on which certain power battles are being played. It would be a mistake to ignore the power element. Until power issues get resolved, resolution of other issues is likely to be temporary at best.

If the safest place for a woman to be is in a relatively equal power balance with her relationship partner (whether that partner is a man or another woman), how best can such a balance be achieved?

Dual Careers

More women than ever before, including mothers of young children, are in the work force. And more than ever before, couples are juggling work roles and family roles. Yet many questions remain about how to help sustain intimate relationships within the context of so much juggling.

The term *dual career* refers to couples in which each partner has a job or career or profession that offers intrinsic rewards, requires substantial training or education as well as highly motivated involvement, and offers opportunities for advancement as well as professional and personal growth. This type of couple can be contrasted with the *dual earner* couple, in which both spouses are employed in jobs with fixed parameters of hours, involvement, advancement, and growth. Finally, the *two-person career* refers to a career in which one spouse (traditionally the husband) occupies an executive position that requires a virtual full-time commitment from the other spouse (traditionally the wife). Such an arrangement offers "two for the price of one." Whatever the terms used, increasing numbers of families have both spouses working, and over 50% of married women who have young children are now in the work force. So the issues are real. This chapter focuses on dual career couples, but the issues generalize to nearly all couples in which both partners are employed.

Some of the central questions for dual career couples have remained unchanged over the years. Whose career comes first? Who takes care of the children? Who grocery shops? But the issues have now become more legitimate targets for negotiation between relationship partners. A decade or two ago, society as a whole, particularly men, questioned the need for women (at least mothers) to work outside the home at all. The economic realities of the past decade, whether plant closings, failed banks, company downsizing, or just the rising cost of living, have made dual incomes a necessity for many families. (And, of course, for millions of single-parent families or single individuals, "not working" has never been an option.) Although not every family makes the choice to have both partners employed, society is not so puzzled today by the families who do. There are fewer "why" questions and more "how" questions regarding the dual career family form.

Men Speak: How Do You Fold the Sheets?

One couple's metaphor for the clash between traditional and egalitarian gender roles (not to mention the shifting power balance) is displayed in a husband's innocent question: "How do you fold the sheets?" Contained in that simple communication (which could just as well refer to cooking, food shopping, or dusting) are a number of metacommunications, including "I've never done this before" ("My mother always did it") or "I'm afraid I'll do it wrong" ("I don't see why I have to do it"). The basic message here is that just when the rules for how men and women would relate to each other seemed fairly clear, the rules changed. And now many people are not quite sure what the rules are in any particular situation. Even some very open-minded men don't know how to fold sheets—and don't want to learn.

In earlier years of dual career couples, men were described as "helping" women with housework. More recently, men have substantially increased their involvement with both child care and housework (Pleck, 1985), although the apportionment is far from equal. Some research has indicated that men's lives have been negatively influenced by their partner's career involvement, especially when this involvement shifts family responsibilities to men. However, a review of relevant research found that husbands were not affected negatively by greater household participation (Menaghan & Parcel, 1990). Indeed, the quality of men's family roles—both marital roles and parental roles—is strongly and positively related to men's general mental health (Barnett, Marshall, & Pleck, 1992). Although folding sheets may not be therapeutic in and of itself, men's family involvement can be therapeutic.

Women Speak: Why Don't You Fold Them Right?

Another part of this couple's metaphor speaks to a wife's desire to "have it both ways." A wife may want her husband to participate equally with her in household work; she also wants him to do it "right." So sometimes she criticizes his way of doing things, and sometimes she does the task herself. Part of what operates here is undoubtedly some need for control, but part is also based on women feeling overly responsible for what goes on at home. (Women even take greater responsibility for marital problems [Hendrick, 1981].) Because women do feel particularly responsible for family welfare, husbands' attitudes toward wives' careers are very important (Thomas, Albrecht, & White, 1984). It is easy to look at the issue of women wanting things done "right" and criticize women for being controlling. However, the other part of the housework tug-of-war is the convenient helplessness that men can project when they do not want to perform a particular task.

Some women end up settling for verbal support of their careers rather than participatory involvement by men in child-rearing and housework. Although men are more involved in these areas than they used to be, they are still much less involved than women. Blumstein and Schwartz (1983) interviewed couples regarding an array of relationship and other concerns. They found that in families where wives worked outside the home, wives still bore the major share of responsibility for housework. Indeed, Hochschild (1989) found that women in dual earner households put in the equivalent of an extra month of labor each year to maintain the household.

Why don't women make more fuss about their disproportionate household burden? As mentioned earlier, women may take this greater burden as a matter of course. However, it also appears that although men are far from carrying an equal share of the household burden (Berardo, Shehan, & Leslie, 1987), a belief that the distribution of labor is "fair" rather than "equal" may be what is needed for relationship success, at least right now. Rachlin (1987) studied dual career and dual earner couples and found that although wives reported more role overload than did husbands, what appeared to contribute to marital adjustment was a "perception" of equity or fairness in the relationship, not necessarily precise equality. So, as is true in many other areas of life, perceptions of the truth may be more important than the "truth" itself.

What We Want versus What We Get

Perhaps one of the greatest areas for partner conflict involves a discrepancy between the family ideal and the family reality. McHale and Crouter (1992) found that couples at greatest risk for less positive marital quality were "wives with nontraditional sex-role attitudes but traditional family work roles and husbands with traditional attitudes but egalitarian roles" (p. 537). It appeared to be less a matter of what each partner had than of how what they had compared to what they wanted. The discrepancy between real and ideal can be very powerful.

As discussed earlier in the section on power and violence, there may be greater risk for violence in a couple where the man feels a power disadvantage. However, a man's gender role attitudes, including traits of both assertiveness and sensitivity, appear to moderate the effect of wives' higher earnings or higher occupational status on husbands' marital quality (Vannoy & Philliber, 1992). In other words, if the husband really believes in gender equality, it will not create problems for her to be more "successful" than he is; it might even be a plus.

It is interesting that while everyone eagerly queries men's gender-related attitudes, women's attitudes are often taken for granted. And research has focused only on how women's employment has had an impact on men, with relatively little attention to the impact of men's employment on women (Menaghan & Parcel, 1990). Maybe that will come later.

Dual career and dual earner families are actors in a drama that highlights issues of changing gender roles and shifting power balances. Of course, sometimes the roles are not changing and sometimes the balances are not shifting, and that itself may be the presenting problem. Couples seldom walk into a therapist's office saying, "We're a dual career couple, and we need help." Instead, they may come in with physical complaints due to stress, conflict because of role strain, disillusionment because the marriage has no romance left, and so on. However, the realities of being in a dual career situation are at best stressful and at worst likely to exacerbate otherwise normal stresses and conflicts. So it is probably wise for a therapist to initially assess the partners' strategies for coping with dual careers. Gilbert (1988) describes three coping strategies for the stress engendered by dual careers: understanding, management, and change. If the woman in a dual career (but also fairly traditional) family finds that early evening is especially hectic because of dinner preparation, she might adopt an *understanding strategy* that would involve accepting the fact that this is a hectic time, that dinner might not always be as good as she'd like, and so on. If she adopts a *management strategy*, she will begin doing some meal preparation on the weekends so the week is a little less hectic. If she embraces a *change strategy*, however, she is likely to negotiate with her husband and children for a new and different division of the cooking responsibilities for the family. All three strategies are adaptive for people at various times, and therapy is an ideal place in which to try out new strategies. Even though the world of heterosexual dual career couples is terribly demanding, that of gay and lesbian couples is even more complicated.

Special Concerns of Gay and Lesbian Couples

Couples are couples in most respects, and lesbian and gay couples encounter most of the problems of heterosexual couples. However, many of these problems are exacerbated by our society's homophobia (Morin, 1977). As noted in an earlier chapter, gay couples typically cohabit because legal marriage is denied them, and it is simply more complicated for gay men and lesbians to establish long-term partnerships (Berzon, 1988).

In addition, gay men and lesbians face some unique problems in the workplace. As Gilbert (1993) points out in her recent volume on dual career families, many employers are still reluctant to extend health and other benefits to same-sex partners of employees. The general working atmosphere also often contributes to a conspiracy of silence about sexual preference such that in one study, two-thirds of the working women had not told their employers they were lesbian, and over one-third said no one in their work setting knew they were lesbian (Eldridge & Gilbert, 1990).

The household sharing that can be such a source of inequity and dissatisfaction to heterosexual couples may be just as troublesome to lesbian and gay male couples, even though tasks are not assigned based on traditional gender division (Berzon, 1988). Household work still needs to be done, however it is "assigned."

Child-rearing complexities are especially difficult for gay and lesbian couples, who are largely discouraged from becoming parents. As Gilbert (1993) points out, the "how" of having children is more complicated for these couples, as is the use of health benefits. The dual career family, particularly the family with children, needs a lot of network support, and "lesbian and gay male couples tend to derive less support from their parents and other family members and to rely more on friendship networks than do married heterosexual couples" (Gilbert, 1993, p. 123).

A therapist dealing with a lesbian or gay male couple needs to be aware of potential within-relationship factors such as power that are significant for any couple, but the therapist must also be sensitized to the added stresses placed on this couple by kinship networks and work settings as well as by the legal system and society as a whole.

Today's close relationships must confront changing gender roles, shifting power balances, and the stresses of two careers, all of which are shown in the following case example.

❧ *Case Example* ❧

Jennifer and Chuck are in their early forties. They have been married for 20 years and have two children, both now in high school. Chuck is the manager of a supermarket, and Jennifer is a secretary. Although Jennifer had been at home with the children while they were small, she had gone back into the work force (with Chuck's encouragement) about ten years ago. For the past couple of years, Jennifer and Chuck have become increasingly unhappy due to Jennifer wanting Chuck to assume more household and family responsibilities. Chuck has resisted taking on more work, and the two have begun arguing. Conflict is what brought them into counseling, where they have already had several sessions. Their "homework" for the past week was to have a cleaning service clean their house.

Therapist: So how have things been?
Jennifer: Better, I guess. At least we haven't been fighting about who's going to clean the bathroom or who's going to vacuum.
Chuck: Yeh, it was nice not to have her (gesturing toward Jennifer) hassling me. I even got to watch some of the play-off games. But we can't afford to do this every week.
Therapist: It sounds like the crisis intervention strategy worked pretty well. But I understand that you don't

believe this will work for the long haul. How did you
spend the time you saved by not cleaning—and not arguing about cleaning?

Chuck: Like I said, I watched some games. And one night the
four of us went out to a movie.

Jennifer: We really didn't do a whole lot. I was glad to be
able to just sit for a while in the evening. Also, I got
caught up on the ironing and even managed to write a
couple of letters.

[Chuck has had more power in the home and felt entitled
to relax, while Jennifer kept working her second shift.]

Therapist: It sounds like this week was definitely better and
that you two used the time pretty well. But Jennifer, it
sounds like your work never quite all gets taken care of.
So, have you two talked about some possible ways of handling this issue?

Chuck: I think we should just make the kids clean the house.
They could do it on the weekend.

Jennifer: Of course that's what you want. They can clean on
Saturday, when you're at the store all day, and that way
you don't have to be involved at all.

Chuck: You always say that. But I help around the house
more than a lot of guys I know.

Jennifer: I know, I know.

Therapist: Chuck, I think that's an important thing you just
said. You said that you "help" around the house. And Jennifer, you agreed. One of the things I find with a lot of
couples where both partners have full-time jobs is that
both people get pretty involved with the kids, if there are
kids, whether it's taking care of little ones or transporting
older ones to activities. But this sharing kind of breaks
down when it comes to housework. Usually it is more the
wife's responsibility to take care of the house, and the
husband "helps." That's not wrong, but it may not be fair.
But I know that you two grew up in families where the
moms stayed at home and the dads didn't do housework,
and where it was pretty clear what women did and what
men did. The rules have changed right in the middle of
the game, and it takes time to get used to new rules.

[Therapist raises awareness of traditional gender roles.]

Chuck: And I haven't gotten used to them yet. Not all of
them. It just never seems to stop. There's always work to
do, either at the store or at home. I get tired of it.

Jennifer: I do too. But somebody's got to do it.

> [Chuck expresses a bit of entitlement, and Jennifer feels responsible.]

Therapist: For some of the work, that's true, but there is some amount of housework that may not have to be done, at least not every week or even every month. And it doesn't necessarily need to be done well. You two may have grown up with a clean house and a hot meal on the table every night (both nod affirmatively). Well, many families can't manage that anymore, and there's no rule that says they have to. There are some alternate ways of handling this and some shortcuts that your family can take. But the first step is not agreeing what you are going to do, it is agreeing "how you are going to agree on what you are going to do." Jennifer, if you decide, and Chuck just "helps" decide, then you're going to have problems.

> [Therapist reframes issue of housework to issue of making a decision, more acceptable to Chuck and less activating of gender role issues.]

Jennifer: I almost don't care what we do if we can just work on it equally as a team. I end up feeling so responsible for the house, and then I feel angry, and then I nag Chuck, and then I feel guilty.

Therapist: Maybe you could make a joint decision.

> [Therapist introduces idea of equal power.]

Chuck: I'm willing to try to share in this. I just don't want to spend all my time at home cleaning toilets or wearing an apron.

Therapist: Okay, let's talk about some of your options.

The therapist goes on to talk with Jennifer and Chuck about a variety of options, ranging from budgeting for monthly cleaning from a cleaning service to hiring (not forcing) the kids to clean the house to cleaning the house as a family. An additional part of the discussion involved the couple's increasing sense of "permission" that they could cut some corners and could do things differently from the way their own families had done them. Developing their own family patterns (rather than trying to superimpose new egalitarian "shoulds" on top of old traditional "shoulds") made the process of change more acceptable to both Chuck and Jennifer.

Summary

Contemporary couples, whether dual career, dual earner, or traditional, whether homosexual or heterosexual, do not have it easy. Evolving gender roles mean that often the old, familiar rules no longer apply. More women are in the labor force, and fewer are full-time homemakers caring for house and children. Society has been slow to recognize the needs of dual career and dual earner families, so pressure often exists on men to "do more" and on women to "do it all." Indeed, men have increased their involvement with both housework and child care; however, women still carry most of the burden.

One issue for many couples is power—who has it under what circumstances? Men have traditionally had more power than have women, at least in the ways in which our culture measures power (for example, resources). Men have used more direct influence strategies and women more indirect ones, though recent research indicates that if men and women have similar amounts of power, they use similar (direct) strategies. Violence is an all too frequent occurrence in couples, and it is directly linked to power. It appears that the safest position for women in heterosexual relationships is to have power equal to that of their partner, no more and no less. One way for women to gain greater power is to be involved in the world of work and be part of a dual career/dual earner couple.[*]

---

[*]As I conclude this chapter, I am hopeful. Within my mother's lifetime, women's right to vote has been made law. Within my lifetime, women's right to equality in the workplace has been made law. Within my daughter's lifetime, women have begun to make the law.

CHAPTER SIX

Transforming Relationships

No one could understand it when Louise and George separated and filed for divorce. What happened? Perhaps they were not the perfect couple (Louise managed to be dependent and controlling at the same time, and George was a bit authoritarian), but they didn't seem to have any major problems. And after all, they had three grown children and had been married for 35 years! Everyone assumed that one of them (probably George) was having an affair (probably with a younger woman), but that didn't prove to be the case. Gradually, as Louise and George began to talk more openly with their friends and family, it became clear that here were two people who had stayed locked in a familiar pattern for much longer than either would have envisioned. Marrying young, they had come together because of love but had stayed together first because of mutual commitment to their children, later because of society's negative sanctions toward divorced persons, and still later because of inertia and the comfort of even uncomfortable familiarity.

This story is repeated every hour of every day, with characters of different ages, from different socioeconomic, ethnic, racial, and religious groups, and with different variations on the central themes. Sometimes there is a quiet, anesthetized disengagement, but all too often there is anger and violence, and nearly always pain.

Although severing romantic relationships includes many examples besides divorce (relationship breakup, death of a partner), it is divorce that has claimed the major portion of attention from the media and from the professionals. Consistent with that emphasis, the primary concern addressed in this chapter is divorce and remarriage counseling (though much of the material is relevant to relationship breakup more generally).

Dialectical Issues:
The Only Stability Is Change

An inherent reality of close romantic relationships is that they are dialectical. Change is the basic tenet of dialectics, and relationships are always changing. Although too much change may induce relationship chaos, extreme resistance to change will eventually wither a relationship. People who do not want to change deny the realities of maturation, aging, and personal growth. Children grow up and leave home. Our jobs change; companies reorganize—or close. Some friends move away. The neighborhood begins to deteriorate. Or sometimes, the neighborhood gets "older," and then young families move in and start the cycle all over again. The basic reality of any relationship is ever-changing.

Dialectical concepts can apply specifically to the relationship disengagement process (Cupach, 1992) and include: (1) autonomy-connection (how dependent versus independent will partners be?), (2) openness-closedness (how much disclosure versus privacy will partners have?), and (3) novelty-predictability (how many unknowns versus knowns do partners want?). These dimensions are handled in different ways at different times in the life of a relationship, and they may also assume differential importance in different relationship stages.

Louise and George maintained some measure of flexibility in these dimensions for the early years of their marriage, but as time went on, the partners remained increasingly at one pole of the dialectic. They became extremely independent, with George preoccupied with business concerns and Louise pouring her energy into family and friends as well as into her work. A natural corollary of autonomy was closedness. Although they had never been intense communicators, George and Louise came to the point where they had little to say to each other beyond chitchat about the house, the dog, and the children and their families. Not surprisingly, predictability was a hallmark of their married life; novelty had no place in their interaction.

Interestingly, dialectical processes operate at several separate but related levels: individual, dyadic, and network (Cupach, 1992). This was clearly the case for Louise and George, who each struggled separately with their personal needs even though the relationship itself seemed stuck. For example, George was never comfortable with the autonomy messages with which he had been raised. He could settle into a relatively traditional position, with modest connectedness taking a clear second position to autonomy. Then his needs for closeness and intimacy would almost overwhelm him, and he would want to get much closer to Louise. For her part, Louise never felt that she knew what to expect from George, so she settled on "autonomy with minimal connection" as the safest place for her to stay emotionally. Her own needs for intimacy and connection were met with family and friend relationships outside the marriage.

These characteristic ways of handling both individual and dyadic dialectics were apparent during the divorce process, when George would coldly and systematically work out with Louise the details about how they were going to divide their property and then later tearfully call her, wanting to get together to "talk things over." There was for him at least a slight wish to reconnect with Louise and reinvest in the marriage, but Louise, feeling that these were just the same mixed messages she'd been hearing from George for years, chose to maintain her autonomy and continue with the divorce process.

The dialectic of opposites—and ideally the transcendence of opposites—is present in all close relationships. "Individuals want to be open and honest, but they also want to protect their partner and preserve their own self-image. They want passion and abandonment but not without security and order" (Cupach, 1992, p. 128). They want—but cannot have—it all. One inevitability in intimate relationships is change.

Perspectives on Relationship Breakup

Raquel and Tom could never agree on anything. They met in a college political science class—Raquel was conservative, and Tom was liberal. Initially, they only disagreed about politics. As they learned more about each other, however, they found that they also disagreed about religion, sports, movies, and even food. Everyone was surprised when the two of them got married; no one was surprised three years later when they got divorced.

Reasons for Breakup

There are almost as many reasons for relationship breakup as there are persons in relationships, but Duck (1982) has proposed three classes of reasons that may lead to dissolution that provide a useful classification system for therapists. The first of these is *pre-existing doom*, and this is what was apparent for Tom and Raquel, almost from the time they first met. Pre-existing doom means that partners are so ill-matched that the relationship never really has any chance for success. The second class of reasons, *mechanical failure/process loss*, refers to partners' inability to be intimate, to communicate, and in general to do those things necessary to keep a relationship going. The final class, *sudden death*, refers to cataclysmic events such as extramarital affairs or other betrayals of trust (for example, one partner has surgery, and the other partner is nowhere to be found).

These three classes of reasons can account for many of the relationship breakups seen by therapists. Couples like Raquel and Tom, who disagree about everything, or who have no common attitudes or values, or who cannot bridge a cultural or racial gap, or who are simply too young and inexperienced to make a relationship commitment, bear the burden of pre-existing doom. George and Louise experienced an erosion of relationship positives and a rigidifying of behaviors at one or the other poles of the various dialectical processes operating in their relationship. They really exemplify the inexorable deadening that comes in the wake of mechanical failure/process loss. Major disruptive relationship experiences (the sudden-death phenomenon) do indeed end relationships, but they are not the predominant destructor of romance. Kurdek (1991) surveyed gay and lesbian partners who had recently broken off long-term close relationships. Not surprisingly, he found that the reasons given for breakup were very similar to those offered by heterosexual partners, as reported in the current literature. The top five reasons given for breakup were: "frequent absence," "sexual incompatibility," "mental cruelty," "lack of love," and "infidelity" (p. 270). Only the fifth reason is a sudden-death phenomenon; the others seem largely to represent mechanical failure/process loss.

As Kurdek (1991) found, a relationship behavior that can lead directly to breakup is infidelity. One partner becomes romantically and sexually involved with another person and begins investing emotional (and sometimes tangible) resources in that relationship. The other partner feels angry, hurt, betrayed, threatened, and so on. Some people focus outward and have jealous rages; others focus inward and get depressed. Although reasons for having an affair are variable, recent research indicates that dissatisfaction with the current relationship is a motivator for women but not for men to have affairs. Women and men had affairs at approximately the same rates, but only for women were these tied to relationship dissatisfaction (Prins, Buunk, & VanYperen, 1993).

Omission versus Commission

Relationships may break up either because certain things happened or because certain other things didn't happen. In past years, "sins of commission" such as alcohol or other abuses were cited as reasons for breakup and divorce (Kaslow & Schwartz, 1987). More recently, "sins of omission" (such as value differences and inability to communicate) cause partners to separate (Albrecht, Bahr, & Goodman, 1983). Framing partners' difficulties as sins of commission versus sins of omission can be useful to both therapist and clients because it has direct implications for interventions that decrease certain partner behaviors and increase other behaviors.

Implications for Therapy

Depending on whether partners are dealing with reasons of pre-existing doom, mechanical failure/process loss, or sudden death, a therapist may focus differently. If a relationship has never worked really well, infidelity may be the catalyst for breakup. If partners have positive feelings for each other but simply lack skills at communicating or negotiating, a therapist has something to work with. Basic skills of learning to make "I" statements, listening carefully, and letting the partner know that they have been heard and understood can all open up new opportunities for learning to problem solve effectively and putting the relationship back on track. If bridging religious, cultural, or racial differences has been the problem, strategies for setting personal and relationship boundaries and avoiding overinvolvement with family and friends (who may disapprove of the relationship) can give partners both the skills and the permission to put their relationship first. For these couples, pre-existing doom may be in the eye of the beholder. In some cases, however, the therapist can best help the partners to be more skillful at dissolving the relationship than they have been at maintaining it.

Couples who have "lost" what they once had may represent a therapist's greatest challenge. A key element in therapy is finding out whether the positives have merely been misplaced or whether they have been lost forever. It takes a while to find this out. One way to begin to assess this is to ask partners to tell the story of their relationship (see Chapter 1) from first meeting to the present time. Probably the key element in the process is the level of involvement and affect shown by the two partners. If telling their story seems to cue their memories of why they got together in the first place and to stir up some of the warmth they once had, the prognosis for the relationship is pretty positive. If, however, there is either a deadening litany of historical events or a combative pursuit of the "true" story, the prognosis is less favorable. Partners experiencing a relationship crisis such as infidelity need to work through the trauma surrounding that specific event before they can begin to deal with broader relationship issues. Anger, feelings of betrayal, guilt, and so on are common, and the therapist-client relationship must include a great deal of trust.

Just as particular forces propel partners toward breakup, other forces serve as barriers to dissolution. Levinger (1979), a longtime relationships researcher, noted that mutual economic investments, fear of children's (and other family members') reactions to dissolution, and social pressure to stay married are all significant barriers to ending a relationship. This perspective is supported by Prins et al. (1993), who found that the major barrier to marital infidelity for both women and men was a personal belief that infidelity is wrong. Thus values proved to be a significant barrier to behavior.

It is apparent that numerous factors propel partners in close relationships toward breakup and divorce, just as other factors restrain the breakup. Therapists will work differently, depending on the relative balance of these factors. For example, if numerous forces are restraining the breakup, the therapist has more flexibility in introducing interventions to improve the relationship. If the propelling forces are quite strong, initial attention will have to be paid to just keeping the partners together (for example, reducing conflict) rather than improving the relationship (for example, increasing communication skills). When the propelling forces simply overwhelm the restraining ones, the result is breakup and divorce.

Separation and Divorce

Dissolving a relationship is not undertaken lightly; in many cases uncertainty and ambivalence characterize movement toward divorce. When counseling partners who are undertaking a divorce, it is important to remember that divorce is not a unitary phenomenon but rather a multifaceted experience. In fact, Bohannan (1970, 1984) proposed six different "types" of divorce: legal divorce (the formal legalities), emotional divorce (the affective part), economic divorce (property arrangements), coparental divorce (custody and related issues), community divorce (dealing with family, friends, and the outside world), and psychic divorce (the final letting go, and moving on to a new life). Although this sounds vaguely like a stage model, it is not. The first five types of divorce occur almost simultaneously; only psychic divorce is clearly a final stage. And even then, two people who have once been bonded together never lose all vestiges of that bonding.

Stages of Breakup

Duck (1982) proposed several phases of the dissolution process, underlining once more that breakup is a process, not an event. He views the process as a movement from the internal to the external, beginning with the *intrapsychic phase*. Here, one partner, Pete, begins to feel negatively about the other partner, Jasmine, and starts considering the costs and benefits of staying in versus getting out of the relationship. At this point, most of the action is in Pete's head; the processes are internal. Unless Pete somehow resolves his dissatisfaction with the relationship or suppresses his feelings (in which case they'll surface again), he and Jasmine move into the *dyadic phase*. There he tells Jasmine about his feelings, she responds, and they begin to struggle with issues of staying together or breaking up. Several different things can happen to halt the process at this point. Pete and Jasmine may work out some of the issues in ways that satisfy both of them (Jasmine's weight gain bothers Pete, but upsets Jasmine herself even more. Jasmine decides to begin an exercise/nutrition program and feels much better about herself. Pete is satisfied). More often, Jasmine would become tearful and angry when confronted by Pete about her weight, reacting with such intensity that Pete backs off. The relationship regains an uneasy homeostasis, but again, Pete's feelings are likely to resurface. When they do so, he and Jasmine again engage in dyadic work but ultimately decide that their various differences defy resolution. They then enter the *social phase*. Here they begin the formal process of dissolution and divorce and go about dealing with the central and peripheral people in their social network. They create what Duck (1982) calls the "face-saving/blame-placing stories and accounts" of their breakup (Pete says he isn't attracted to Jasmine anymore; they aren't compatible. Jasmine says Pete is immature and doesn't know how to be truly intimate in a relationship.) Finally, they move into the *grave-dressing phase* in which they go through the rituals of mourning the dead relationship and then dress or decorate the grave with stories about the "what weres" and the "could have beens."

Researchers have found that the partner more likely to be willing to leave a relationship (Pete, in the example above) is the one who is less dependent on it in the sense of feeling that important needs are being satisfied (Drigotas & Rusbult, 1992). The "leaving" partner is also the one who feels greater options for having those needs satisfied in one or more alternative relationships. This confirms therapists' experience with numerous couples in which one partner clearly had more to lose in a relationship breakup and was struggling (in vain) to hold onto the partner. This research also accounts for cases that puzzle therapists—cases where "people sometimes remain involved in relationships with apparent serious deficiencies. Such a relationship may persist because the deficiency concerns a need that is less central to that relationship, because the relationship compensates for the deficiency by fulfilling other important needs, or because the meager level of fulfillment nevertheless exceeds what is available elsewhere" (Drigotas & Rusbult, 1992, p. 86).

Looking back at Duck's (1982) four stages of breakup, it appears that clients enter therapy in each of the four stages. When a person in individual therapy focuses primarily on their marital dissatisfaction but their partner "won't" come to therapy, that may be someone in the intra-psychic phase who does not want their partner in the therapy room. Pete might see a therapist because of depression but then spend a whole session complaining about Jasmine's obesity and unappealingness. Couples in the dyadic phase may be experiencing much conflict as well as some estrangement, but they are in a good position to make changes. Jasmine and Pete could feel much safer working on his issues of dissatisfaction and her issues of rejection in the presence of a supportive therapist. Unfortunately, many couples don't see a therapist until they are in the social phase. They may have already talked with their families and friends and may have even had a preliminary meeting with an attorney. For example, Pete and Jasmine may have already started their public accounts of their disengagement: "She's fat and won't take care of herself" and "He's selfish and immature." However, they can be supported in putting this process on hold, at least until they try seriously to resolve their issues.

If either Pete or Jasmine comes in during the grave-dressing phase saying, "I'm in the process of getting a divorce; I need help to cope with it," the therapist will focus on quite different things. To deal with feelings of anger and depression, Jasmine might begin an exercise program, start keeping a journal, join a support group. Pete might begin paying attention to his own health, reconnect with his two sisters, join a therapy group. When someone comes to therapy because of a possible or actual breakup or divorce, a therapist can try to ascertain what stage of the process they are in.

Consequences of Divorce

When people write about divorce, they tend to overwhelm the reader with statistics. However, whether one out of two or one out of three marriages ends in divorce, broken relationships are everywhere. Consequences of divorce vary greatly depending on financial arrangements, presence or absence of children, and so on. But some general and fairly predictable outcomes impinge directly on therapy with a divorcing client.

Health.   Divorce is a major stressor, and clients need to monitor their health during and after divorce. Bloom, Asher, and White (1978) documented links between separation and divorce and such negative health events as higher rates of physical and psychiatric illness, and increased rates of auto accidents and alcoholism. Marital disruption has also been linked to suicide and homicide. Although more recent research (Burman & Margolin, 1992) does not confirm tight links between divorce and health problems, and though most people do not experience such dramatic negative effects, any stressful period is a time for consistent exercise, good nutrition, adequate sleep, and maintaining or in some cases renewing connections to social network supports.

Economics.   A major stressor of divorce is economic problems. Both men and women clients are likely to experience financial problems during divorce, but on average, women will hurt more economically (Barber & Eccles, 1992; Kitson & Morgan, 1990). Women without effective work skills are particularly disadvantaged. Even if an ex-husband pays adequate support, this kind of economic dependency has its price. Divorced women with adequate work skills make at least some economic recovery over time, however (Peterson, 1989).

Two of the couples presented earlier in the chapter represent very different examples of the economics of divorce. When George and Louise divorced, George agreed to a substantial financial settlement that would give Louise their house and provide a modest income for her until she reaches retirement age. Although Louise has a job she likes, it is one without much growth potential in either status or salary. So the settlement was needed. If Pete and Jasmine were to divorce, however, the situation could be different. Jasmine has a good job as a high school teacher, and Pete is a successful salesman. A no-fault divorce would mean that Jasmine would get no alimony and only modest child support for their two grade-school-age children. If Pete indeed pays the support, Jasmine could probably manage financially, though Pete would have a considerably higher income. If he does not pay support, Jasmine and the children would struggle.

Women and children have a right to economic survival after divorce. Therapists working with women in these situations can provide support, empowerment, and strategies. Women may need to acquire education or training, get jobs or make job changes, sue for back child support, and so on. Men may need particular understanding as they work to maintain a connected relationship with their children, if they do not have custody. Active, behavioral-oriented strategies are likely to be helpful during this high stress crisis period. Intra-psychic, exploratory approaches may work better once a woman is sure she can pay her mortgage payment or a man feels confident that he can stay involved with his children.

Children.   The welfare of children during and after divorce is one of the most important concerns of many researchers; and certainly therapists who work with children are well aware of the disruption that divorce can cause. Different reactions occur depending on the child's age and life stage (Santrock & Sitterle, 1987). Preschoolers may be confused and fearful, blaming themselves. Play therapy and supportive interventions are helpful. Young school-age children (6 to 8 years) may be better able to express feelings yet still be confused. Again, play and supportive therapy can help. Older children (9 to 12 years) and adolescents may have divided loyalties and greater anger. For these age groups, supportive therapy, behavioral strategies for coping with the divorce and staying connected but not overinvolved with each parent, and peer support groups can all aid in the recovery process. Although social interactions and school work may be affected, disruptions lessen greatly over a two-year span (Hetherington, 1987).

Parents' abilities to handle the divorce are a key to children's divorce recovery. Authoritative (warm, clear rules, good communication) parenting and maintenance of at least a civil relationship between the parents help children to prosper (Hetherington, 1987; Lowery & Settle, 1985).

In terms of custody issues, joint custody is becoming more common, though it is not without problems (Kitson & Morgan, 1990). There has been a perception that children who are in single-parent families do better when the family is headed by a same-sex parent (that is, girls do better with mom, and boys with dad), but recent research indicates that "for youths in early adolescence, the consequences of living with a same-sex parent are not noticeably different from living with an opposite-sex parent" (Downey & Powell, 1993, p. 68). Although the findings on a number of issues are unclear, therapists can be fairly sure that by helping ex-spouse parents to reduce their overt conflicts; heal their own wounds; avoid triangulating the children; ensure the children's financial welfare; and maintain frequent, positive contact with the children; children's recovery after divorce will be fostered.

Adult recovery.   Although there are a number of ways to help adult clients through the divorce-recovery process, a recent perspective differentiates recovery in terms of (1) reaction to breakup and (2) recovery itself (Frazier & Cook, 1993). Initial reaction to a breakup was more distressed when there was greater satisfaction with a partner, when the relationship had been closer, and when it seemed less likely that another partner could be found (note similarities to Drigotas & Rusbult, 1992). However, recovery from a breakup was greater when there was good social support and when the individual had higher self-esteem. Therapists need to be aware that clients who show the greatest upset at the time of divorce are not necessarily those who will have the rockiest recovery. Clients with healthy self-esteem/ego strength and a strong social support system are likely to have better recoveries.

A postscript.   Much has been written about divorce, and more is probably on its way. The very frequency with which divorce occurs makes it almost a normative event in some people's eyes. For other people, however, this normative tendency is frightening, and in recent months there has been a resurgence of voices urging couples to "stay together for the sake of the children." This may well be a divorce backlash, and it may continue.

A therapist's job is not to judge clients nor to tell them what to do. Rather, it is to help them make the best choices they can and to forgive themselves along the way. Divorce is part of the social fabric. Society is continually reinventing itself, responding to dialectical tensions in the same ways in which individuals and relationships do. Although divorce is disruptive and frightening on one level, it is a part of the ongoing social transformation characteristic of any thriving society. Another part of that transformation is remarriage and blended families.

Remarriage and Blended Families

Shelley and Ted had been married for six months. Each had been married previously, and each had custody of their children (Ted's daughters were 11 and 15; Shelley's daughter was 10 and her son 7). The partners had been introduced by mutual friends, fallen in love quickly, and married after a rather short courtship. They realized that the new "family" would take some adjusting to, but they loved each other very much and believed that things would work out. They had not reckoned with the children's resistance, not so much to the marriage but rather to the family constellation. So after six months of children's whining and crying, sibling and stepsibling fights, and their own frustration and increasing hostility toward each other, Shelley and Ted both believed that they needed help. The problems they brought into therapy were neither unusual nor particularly complex; they were simply problems requiring novel rather than traditional solutions. During both couple and family sessions, Ted and Shelley received therapist support to nurture their own relationship, whether or not things were going smoothly with the children at that particular time. Each parent was encouraged to take the lead in disciplining their own biological children, letting the stepparent ease into things. The children were each given their own "space" in the house and not expected to immediately form one big happy family. The whining and fights were put into perspective (the kids were all doing fine in school, and they even got along together a good share of the time) so that family life could be reframed as "pretty good most of the time but interrupted by fights and disruptions" rather than "awful and not at all what we'd expected." The therapist helped the family normalize their experience, reduce expectations, and be more patient with themselves and each other.

The thinking about remarriage and remarried families has evolved along with terminology. "Stepfamily" sometimes conjured up images of wicked stepmothers or stepfathers—kind of a Cinderella phenomenon. "Blended family" seemed to imply a perfect arrangement in which everyone just naturally got along and lived happily ever after. The current term, "remarried family," really just describes the reality of the situation without making assumptions. These families are increasingly common, and perhaps a third of all children will be part of such a family during their growing up (Fursten-berg, 1987). Remarried families experience all the stresses of intact families and a few additional ones, but the extent to which intact and remarried famlies are similar or different is often not captured by current research approaches. (For an excellent review, see Coleman and Ganong, 1990.)

One important point is the great diversity within remarried families. These range from families with only one previously married spouse with children, to families with both spouses previously married with children, to spouses involved in several remarriages or "serial marriage" (Brody, Neubaum, & Forehand, 1988). In each of these situations, dynamics and problems are likely to be somewhat different. Counseling with remarried families requires a thorough assessment of the family's history.

Although remarried couples and families may come into therapy with the same issues that bring other people (for example, wife's depression, adolescent's acting out), remarried families have some unique concerns. One major problem is negative "myths" (though overly positive myths can be a problem also). Remarried families are the stuff of which fairy tales such as "Snow White" and "Hansel and Gretel" are made, and it is tough to combat images so embedded in socialization. Stepmothers often fare even worse than stepfathers in the myth-making process, probably because the expectations for nurturing are higher for women than for men in this society (Goldenberg & Goldenberg, 1990).

But roles are not easy for stepfathers either. Men often do not have custody of their biological children, so they may be weekend Dads with their own children, weekday Dads with their stepchildren, and then feel torn in the process. And the children, who did not really have much choice about this life-style, are many times mourning their old life while trying to adjust to their new one.

Overall, those who work with remarried families realize that these families can work wonderfully well under the right circumstances. In fact, remarried couples are likely to be just as or more satisfied than ever-married couples when total family functioning is not considered (Anderson & White, 1986). And Smith (1992) found that family cohesion in remarried and intact families was quite similar except where the remarried families had adolescents.

There have been a number of ways of looking at remarried families (Coleman & Ganong, 1990). These include the *socialization hypothesis* (children in remarried families may be less adequately socialized); the *biological-discrimination hypothesis* (stepparents may have less parental investment in stepchildren than in biological children), and the *incomplete-institution hypothesis* (the stepfamily is not a "real" family). More recently, the normative-adaptive perspective has abandoned earlier deficit, pathology-focused models and recognizes divorce and remarriage as life-style choices that need to be accepted and analyzed rather than judged. As this perspective gains hold, issues such as the legal rights of stepparents and stepchildren (payment of child support, custody, and visitation) are likely to receive increasing attention (Fine & Fine, 1992). "Although we have focused to a great degree on the problems of remarried families, such families may offer positive benefits to children in the form of an additional extended family and new role models and relationships that can greatly enrich the child's life experience" (Hendrick & Hendrick, 1992a, p. 210).

A number of useful resources are available for remarried families and for therapists who work with them (for example, Coleman & Ganong, 1990; Goldenberg & Goldenberg, 1990; Visher & Visher, 1979, 1988; Walsh, 1992). A classic list of guidelines for remarried families compiled by the Vishers (1979) provides a useful starting point. (See Box 6.1.)

B O X   6.1
Guidelines for Stepfamilies

1. It is difficult to have a new person or persons move into your "space," and it is difficult to be the "new" person or people joining a preexisting group. For these reasons, it helps to cut down feelings involved with "territory" if families can start out in a new house or apartment.

2. Parent-child relationships have preceded the new couple relationship. Because of this, many parents feel that it is a betrayal of the parent-child bond to form a primary relationship with their new partner. A primary couple relationship, however, is usually crucial for the continuing existence of the stepfamily, and therefore is very important for the children as well as for the adults. A strong adult bond can protect the children from another family loss, and it also can provide the children with a positive model for their own eventual marriage relationship. The adults often need to arrange time alone to help nourish this important couple relationship.

3. Forming new relationships within the stepfamily can be important, particularly when the children are young. Activities involving different subgroups can help such relationships grow. For example, stepfather and stepchildren might do some project together; or stepmother and a stepchild might go shopping together.

4. Preserving original relationships is also important and can help children experience less loss at sharing a parent. So at times it is helpful

for a parent and natural children to have some time together, in addition to stepfamily activities.

5. Caring relationships take time to evolve. The expectation of "instant love" between stepparents and stepchildren can lead to many disappointments and difficulties. If the stepfamily relationships are allowed to develop as seems comfortable to the individuals involved, then caring between steprelatives has the opportunity to develop.

6. Subsequent families are structurally and emotionally different from first families. Upset and sadness are experienced by the children and at times by the adults as they react to the loss of their nuclear family or to the loss of a dream of a perfect marriage. Acceptance that a stepfamily is a new type of family is important. It is also very helpful to recognize that this type of family pattern can provide the opportunity for children and adults to grow and mature and lead satisfying lives. Many upsetting behaviors may result from these feelings of insecurity and loss.

7. Because children are part of two biological parents, they nearly always have very strong pulls to both of these natural parents. These divided loyalties often make it difficult for children to relate comfortably to all the parental adults in their lives. Rejection of a stepparent, for example, may have nothing to do with the personal characteristics of the stepparent. In fact, warm and loving stepparents may cause especially severe loyalty conflicts for children. As children and adults are able to accept the fact that children can care for more than two parental adults, then the children's loyalty conflicts can diminish and the new step-relationships improve. While it may be helpful to the children for the adults to acknowledge negative as well as positive feelings about ex-spouses, children may become caught in loyalty conflicts and feel personally insecure if specific critical remarks are made continuously about their other natural parent.

8. Courteous relationships between ex-spouses are important, although they are very difficult for many adults to maintain. If such a relationship can be worked out, it is especially helpful to the children. In such instances, the children do not get caught in the middle between two hostile parents, there is less need for the children to take sides, and the children are better able to accept and utilize the positive elements in the living arrangements.

Direct contact between the adults can be helpful since it does not place the children in the sometimes powerful position of being message carriers between their natural parents. Although it may be strained, many ex-spouses are able to relate in regards to their children if the focus is kept on their mutual concern for the welfare of the children.

9. Children as well as adults in a stepfamily have a "family history." Suddenly these individuals come together and their sets of "givens" are questioned. Much is to be gained by coming together as a stepfamily unit

to work out and develop new family patterns and traditions. During these "family negotiation sessions," the feelings and ideas of all members are important, regardless of age. Many creative solutions can be worked out as a family.

Even when the individuals are able to recognize that patterns are not "right" or "wrong," it takes time and patience to work out satisfying new alternatives. Values (the underlying approach to life in general ways of doing things) do not shift easily. Within a stepfamily, different value systems are inevitable because of different previous family histories, and tolerance for these differences can help smooth the process of stepfamily integration. Needs (specific ways individuals relate together and individual preferences) can usually be negotiated more quickly than can general values. Having an appreciation for and an expectation of such difficulties can make for more flexibility and relaxation in the stepfamily unit. Negotiation and renegotiation are needed by most such families.

10. Being a stepparent is an unclear and at times difficult task. The wicked stepmother myth contributes to the discomfort of many women, and cultural, structural, and personal factors affect the stepparent role. Spouses can be very helpful to one another if they are able to be supportive with the working out of new family patterns. Stepparenting is usually more successful if stepparents carve out a role for themselves that is different from and does not compete with the natural parents.

While discipline is not usually accepted by stepchildren until a friendly relationship has been established (often a matter of 18 to 24 months), both adults do need to support each other's authority in the household. The natural parent may be the primary disciplinarian initially, but when that person is unavailable, it is often necessary for that parent to give a clear message to the children that the stepparent is acting as an "authority figure" for both adults in his or her absence.

Unity between the couple is important to the functioning of the stepfamily. When the couple is comfortable with each other, differences between them in regard to the children can sometimes be worked out in the presence of the children, but at no time does it work out for either children or adults to let the children approach each adult separately and "divide and conquer." When disciplinary action is necessary, if it is not kept within the stepfamily household many resentful feelings can be generated. For example, if visitation rights are affected, the noncustodial parent is being included in the action without his or her representation. Such a punishment, then, may lead to difficulties greater than the original behavior that caused the disciplinary action.

11. Integrating a stepfamily that contains teenagers can be particularly difficult. Adolescents are moving away from their families in any type of family. In single-parent families, teenagers have often been "young adults," and with the remarriage of a parent they may find it

extremely difficult or impossible to return to being in a "child" position again.

Adolescents have more of a previous "family history" and so they ordinarily appreciate having considerable opportunity to be part of the stepfamily negotiations, although they may withdraw from both natural parents and not wish to be part of many of the "family" activities.

12. "Visiting" children usually feel strange and are outsiders in the neighborhood. It can be helpful if they have some place in the household that is their own; for example, a drawer or shelf for toys and clothes. If they are included in stepfamily chores and projects when they are with the stepfamily, they tend to feel more connected to the group. Bringing a friend with them to share the visit and having some active adult participation in becoming integrated into the neighborhood can make a difference to many visiting children. Knowing ahead of time that there is going to be an interesting activity (such as a stepfamily game of Monopoly) can sometimes give visiting children a pleasant activity to anticipate.

Noncustodial parents and stepparents often are concerned because they have so little time to transmit their values to visiting children. Since children tend to resist concerted efforts by the adults to instill stepfamily ideals during each visit, it is comforting to parents and stepparents to learn that the examples of behavior and relationships simply observed in the household can affect choices made by all the children later in their lives when they are grown and on their own.

13. Sexuality is usually more apparent in stepfamilies because of the new couple relationship, and because children may suddenly be living with other children with whom they have not grown up. Also, there are not the usual incest taboos operating. It is important for the children to receive affection and to be aware of tenderness between the couple, but it may also be important for the couple to minimize to some extent the sexual aspects of the household and to help the children understand, accept, and control their sexual attractions to one another or to the adults.

14. All families experience stressful times. Children tend to show little day-to-day appreciation for their parents, and at times they get angry and reject their natural parents. Because stepfamilies are families born of loss, the mixture of feelings can be even more intense than in intact families. Jealousy, rejection, guilt, and anger can be more pronounced, and therefore expectations that the stepfamily will live "happily ever after" are unrealistic. Having an understanding and acceptance of the many negative as well as positive feelings can result in less disappointment and more stepfamily enjoyment.

15. Keeping even minimal contact between adults and children can lead to future satisfaction since time and maturity bring many changes. With some communication between stepfamily members, satisfying

interpersonal relationships often develop in the future when children become more independent in their relationships with both natural parents and with stepparents.

SOURCE: From *Stepfamilies: A Guide to Working with Stepparents and Stepchildren*, by E. B. Visher and J. S. Visher, Copyright 1979 by Brunner/Mazel, Inc. Reprinted by permission.

Issues of relationship formation, dissolution, and reformation are part of all of our lives. In addition to providing endings, divorce and remarriage may also provide beginnings. Some of these issues of relationship transformation are explored in the following case example.

❧ *Case Example* ❧

Nancy and Cliff have been married for five years. This is the second marriage for each of them. Nancy's two children, Kim (age 14) and Jed (age 12), have always lived with Nancy and Cliff except for holiday visits and summer vacations with their biological father, who lives in another state. Cliff's son Tim (age 13) has been living with his mother. After some initial problems, the family unit had functioned extremely well. Cliff and Nancy thought that all the stepfamily issues had been worked out—until Tim came to live with them five months ago. Suddenly the kids were bickering with each other, Kim was starting to question family rules that were well established, Nancy and Cliff had begun arguing about the children, and Tim seemed just generally depressed. Nancy and Cliff were referred for family counseling but expressed interest in working on couple issues first. They are highly motivated and have had several sessions already.

Therapist: So, how have things been this week?

Cliff: Fine. The kids have been really busy with schoolwork, so they haven't had time to argue much.

Nancy: That's not quite true. Kim and Jed have been busy with homework—I'm not sure what Tim has been doing besides playing music so loud it practically shakes the house.

Cliff: (Sitting back in his chair and looking tense and a little down) Yes, I guess you're right.

Therapist: Wait a minute. Do you two know what just happened? (Both shake their heads "No") I asked how things

were going, Cliff said "pretty well," Nancy made a negative comment, and Cliff agreed but then pulled out of the
conversation and back into his chair. That's the kind of
process we've been talking about in here. Cliff says something that may minimize the problem, Nancy reacts with
anger, and Cliff just drops out.

Nancy: I know. I need to keep my mouth shut. I love Cliff; I
don't want him to drop out. I don't want to turn him off
or hurt him. I just feel frustrated by Tim so much of the
time. He's so different from my kids.

Cliff: I hate it when you call Kim and Jed "your kids." They're
my kids too; I love them.

Nancy: I know you do. And I feel so guilty, because I ought to
be able to say that I love Tim—and I can't. (She gets tears
in her eyes)

Therapist: I think that is a key issue right there. Nancy, Cliff
has had five years to form relationships with Kim and
Jed. You've only had five months to try to get acquainted
with Tim. Before, you were just a "vacation mother."
Now, you're his day-in and day-out stepmother. That's
very different. Give yourself some time. There is no "bad
guy" here, just some nice people trying to get a family to
work better.

[Therapist encourages giving selves more time; see #5 in
guidelines for stepfamilies.]

Cliff: That's what I tell her. Tim needs time to get used to
being with us. He doesn't know the rules.

Therapist: And he needs time to learn them—but he does
have to learn them. And he needs to learn them mostly
from you, Cliff. It is important that the stepparent not be
put in the role of the "heavy." You've already told me that
when you were first married, Nancy handled most of the
discipline for Kim and Jed.

[Initially, biological parent needs to do most of disciplining;
see #10 in guidelines for stepfamilies.]

Cliff: I know you're right. I don't like having to be tough with
Tim, but I guess that I have to.

Therapist: I'm not sure that you so much have to be "tough"
as be firm and consistent. It's very important for you to
connect with Tim in several different ways; you'll need to
give some extra time to that relationship for a while.
Maybe you can even explain to Kim and Jed that you will

be giving Tim a little "extra" for a while; they probably will understand.

Nancy: Cliff, if you took more responsibility for Tim, I think that I wouldn't feel so responsible and then get so upset when things don't go the way I think they should. I just feel like it's my fault when we all don't get along better. I don't feel like I'm doing very well with Kim right now, as a matter of fact.

[Gender role issues again, with Nancy feeling responsible for entire family.]

Therapist: That's another area I want to talk with you about. Kim is getting to the age where she's going to start "moving out" of the family space a little. Don't assume that every conflict is because you're a remarried family or because Tim has just come to live with you. Some of these family issues were bound to happen anyway. They're normal.

[Adolescents need to begin individuating, no matter what the family constellation; see #11 of guidelines for step-families.]

Nancy: I feel a little less pressure, hearing you say that. I want to be a good mother, and I certainly don't want to be the "wicked stepmother."

[Family stress is normal; see #14 in guidelines for step-families.]

Cliff: I feel better too, but I know that we still have a lot of work ahead of us.

The session continues, and this couple, and eventually the whole family, continues in therapy for several months. Many of the issues prove to be very difficult, but the therapist's consistent message to the family is from the normative-adaptive perspective and says, "You're okay."

Summary

There is a dialectical nature to close relationships, particularly in such areas as autonomy-connection, openness-closedness, and novelty-predictability. The ability to flexibly accommodate change may indicate whether a relationship continues or terminates.

Relationships end for many reasons, including pre-existing problems, erosion of the quality of the relationship, and traumatic relationship events. Infidelity is one of these traumatic events, though sins of both omission and commission may contribute to a relationship's ending. The divorce process includes legal, emotional, economic, coparental, community, and psychic aspects. In addition, divorce has come to be viewed as a process rather than an event, and as moving through internal, dyadic, social, and mourning phases.

Divorce has health and economic consequences for adults as well as many other consequences for the children involved. Parental coping with divorce is a major factor in children's resilience. Many divorced families become part of remarried families, and these families experience stressors such as myths and loyalty issues. As remarried families come to be viewed as an alternative family form rather than a defective family form, society is likely to become more supportive to these families.

CHAPTER SEVEN

Professional
and Ethical Issues

Jamal had been in the counseling field for a number of years, and much of his work was with couples and families. Leah and Jerry, a married couple in their thirties, had been referred to Jamal because the partners had been discussing divorce, due largely to Leah's dissatisfaction. The first time he met Jerry and Leah, Jamal was a bit startled. Both were pleasant, intelligent people, and Leah was an average-looking (even modestly attractive) woman. However, Jerry, though neat and well-dressed, appeared to be about 100 to 150 pounds overweight. As the partners discussed their relationship across several therapy sessions, Leah never mentioned Jerry's weight as a reason for her decreasing interest in staying in the marriage. Although Jamal introduced the topic several times, Leah only partially acknowledged Jerry's weight as an issue for her. But Jamal kept feeling that it was more of a problem than Leah would admit. However, he also recognized that the topic of weight was one that "pushed his buttons." Jamal had been involved previously with a woman who gained a great deal of weight during the course of their relationship. This was a major turn-off for Jamal and ultimately became one of the factors in their breakup. Thus, he now couldn't help wondering whether Jerry's weight was really a problem for Leah—or was only a problem for Jamal himself.

ಶಿ

Therapists bring their own personalities and life experiences into their work. Current and past personal relationships form a backdrop for relationships with clients, and it is important to be aware of what is influencing the therapeutic direction at any given time. However, the complexity increases when working with a couple. It is necessary to monitor reactions to each partner, to the therapeutic alliance with each partner, and to the relationship itself. It is as though there are three clients: two partners and their relationship.

The close relationships literature has virtually nothing to say about ethics. That is because this literature is preoccupied with theoretical and empirical issues of partnered relationships rather than with the treatment of partners once the relationship develops problems. In some sense, this literature is concerned with prevention issues much more than with remediation issues. Thus, the material in the current chapter is drawn from the more general counseling and marriage and family literatures. This discussion is in no way exhaustive. For excellent in-depth presentations of ethical issues in human service professions see Bennett, Bryant, VandenBos, and Greenwood (1990); Corey, Corey, and Callanan (1993); Keith-Spiegel and Koocher (1985); and Pope and Vasquez (1991).

The primary goals are to introduce some of the major ethical questions confronting those who work with couples and to stimulate new ways of thinking about ethics in relationships—both the therapist's own relationships and those of the clients.

Counseling Couples: Ethical Issues

Couple therapists come from many different disciplines, and different groups have different formal ethical codes. The American Association for Marriage and Family Therapy (AAMFT) Code of Ethics[*] (1991) is one directly linked to working with couples, and its major points can serve as a guideline for discussion.

I. *Responsibility to Clients*: "Marriage and family therapists advance the welfare of families and individuals. They respect the rights of those persons seeking their assistance, and make reasonable efforts to ensure that their services are used appropriately."

This is one of the most important general ethical precepts, because it sets the tone for the therapy relationship. Details of this section of the code state that therapists do not refuse services because of a client's race, gender, religion, national origin, or sexual orientation. Therapists don't engage in dual (that is, personal, professional) relationships with clients; sexual involvement is not permitted for two years following the termination of therapy. Therapists do not prosper at their clients' expense and do not continue therapy longer than

---

[*]Excerpts from the AAMFT Code of Ethics. Copyright 1991, American Association for Marriage and Family Therapy. Reprinted with permission. *No additional copies may be made without obtaining permission from AAMFT.*

necessary. Therapists aid clients in decision making, but the power and the responsibility are the client's. If therapists cannot provide needed treatment, they facilitate treatment for the client elsewhere. Finally, taping, recording, or observing sessions is done only with the client's permission. The client comes first.

II. *Confidentiality*: "Marriage and family therapists have unique confidentiality concerns because the client in a therapeutic relationship may be more than one person. Therapists respect and guard confidences of each individual client."

Therapists break confidentiality only (a) as required by law, (b) when a client represents a danger to self or others, (c) when the therapist is a defendant in a criminal, civil, or disciplinary case, or (d) when appropriate waivers have been signed by all relevant family members. In addition, case material can be used in teaching, writing, and so on only if appropriate client waivers have been signed or the material has been appropriately disguised. Finally, records are stored so as to maintain confidentiality. The security provided by confidentiality is a client right.

III. *Professional Competence and Integrity*: "Marriage and family therapists maintain high standards of professional competence and integrity."

Therapists violate this code if they are convicted of a felony, convicted of a misdemeanor related to their profession, engage in behavior leading to a felony or misdemeanor related to their profession, are disciplined by relevant professional organizations, have licenses revoked, practice therapy while impaired due to substance abuse, or fail to cooperate in the course of an ethical complaint against them. Therapists are expected to behave within ethical and legal standards— period. Therapists also seek help for their own problems. They are accurate in the information they give, stay current in their relevant professional area, try to prevent any misuse of their clinical or research findings, do not practice beyond their areas of competence, and are especially careful when making any public statements. Finally, therapists do not in any way harrass or exploit others. High standards of professional conduct are imperative.

IV. *Responsibility to Students, Employees, and Supervisees*: "Marriage and family therapists do not exploit the trust and dependency of students, employees, and supervisees."

Just as with clients, therapists don't engage in dual relationships with those persons with whom they have a position of relative power— students, supervisees, and employees. Sexual involvement with students and supervisees is not acceptable. Therapists do not allow their students, supervisees, and employees to practice beyond their areas of competence. Finally, therapists do not disclose supervisee confidences except (a) as required by law, (b) when the supervisee represents a danger to self or others, (c) when the therapist is a defendant in a criminal, civil, or disciplinary case, (d) in educational settings only to other involved supervisors, or (e) when an appropriate waiver has been signed. High standards extend to all those with whom a therapist works.

V. *Responsibility to Research Participants*: "Investigators respect the dignity and protect the welfare of participants in research and are aware of federal and state laws and regulations and professional standards governing the conduct of research."

The therapist/researcher observes ethical safeguards in conducting research, employs fully informed consent that is in no way coerced, affords participants the freedom to withdraw from research at any time, and preserves confidentiality for participants unless such rights are waived.

VI. *Responsibility to the Profession*: "Marriage and family therapists respect the rights and responsibilities of professional colleagues and participate in activities which advance the goals of the profession."

Essentially, therapists are expected to be responsible and progressive contributors to their profession and to the wider community that the profession serves. Therapists are accountable. They share publication credit as appropriate, reference appropriately, make sure their authored materials are used correctly, serve their communities (including engaging in pro bono services), promote legislation that serves the public interest, and encourage public involvement in improving professional services. Ethical obligations extend to the wider world.

VII. *Financial Arrangements*: "Marriage and family therapists make financial arrangements with clients, third party payors, and supervisees that are reasonably understandable and conform to accepted professional practices."

Therapists do not pay for or accept payment for referrals. They also charge reasonable fees, disclose those fees before providing services, and are accurate in reporting facts regarding these services.

VIII. *Advertising*: "Marriage and family therapists engage in appropriate informational activities, including those that enable laypersons to choose professional services on an informed basis."

This is the final and most detailed (19 subpoints) of the sections in the ethical code. The first seven points concern "truth in advertising" issues, making certain that any advertising done by a therapist (for example, business cards, stationery, directories, or media advertising) provides enough information for potential consumers to make informed choices about obtaining therapy and contains no false or misleading information. In addition, this truth in advertising must be extended to anyone employed by the therapist. The remaining 12 points in this section are concerned with using AAMFT designations in advertising and offer a number of limitations on advertising format as well as several examples.

Even a brief overview of the basic ethical concerns in marriage and family therapy reveals the complexity of the issues. Ethical choices begin as therapists start their training, before the first client is ever seen, and end with the method for storing and disposing of client records after therapy has terminated. When therapy is chosen as a profession, because of the quasi-public and potentially influential nature of the profession, there are accompanying ethical obligations that extend well past the door of the therapy room. Because ethical issues are so crucially important, therapists are urged to consult their own profession's ethical guidelines, laws in their particular state affecting their profession, and additional resource materials such as Corey et al., (1993).

Related Professional Issues

Although the ethical issues of greatest concern to both supervisees and supervisors are often related to informed consent, assessment of client dangerousness, and other issues that have legal implications (Corey et al., 1993), many of the day-to-day dilemmas for therapists concern the therapist as a "person" relating to another "person" (or persons), the client.

In a survey of practicing therapists, Green and Hansen (1989) found considerable commonality in the types of ethical dilemmas experienced by practicing therapists and developed a list of the 16 most frequent ethical problems. The top five problems, in descending order of occurrence were:

1. Whether to begin treatment without having the entire family in therapy.
2. Holding different values from those of the family.
3. Whether and how to treat the family if one member exits therapy.
4. Professional development for the therapist.
5. Imposing therapist values on the family.

These issues in large measure involve the context of therapy, and they warrant extended discussion.

Who Is the Client? (Numbers 1 and 3)

In the case example that opened this chapter, both marital partners (Leah and Jerry) were committed to couple therapy. But what if Leah had come in alone, citing her increasing dissatisfaction with her marriage as the reason for seeking help? It is likely that Jamal, trained as a couple therapist, would frame Leah's problem as a "couple issue" and would talk to her about getting Jerry to enter couple therapy with her. But what if Leah refuses, saying she wants to work individually? Or what if Jerry refuses to join Leah? Or what if both begin marital treatment, and then one drops out? Some couple therapists require that all relevant members in a couple or family conflict be involved in treatment. Such therapists believe it is at best counter-therapeutic and at worst unethical to see just one individual. However, other couple therapists will work with whoever is willing to participate in therapy, including individuals who represent only part of a couple or family. Both positions can be defended on ethical grounds.

Even if both partners are present in therapy, they may have very different goals. As Corey et al. (1993) ask, when one partner seeks divorce counseling while the other seeks counseling to save the marriage, which partner is the primary client? One approach to this quandry is to make "the relationship" the primary client, believing that with clearer communication and more nurturing and equitable ways of relating to each other, partners will make a better decision about the relationship, whether they stay together or break up.

Therapist Values (Numbers 2 and 5)

Another important area of concern to therapists is the inevitable value clashes that occur in therapy. In their book on counseling families, Goldenberg and Goldenberg (1990) point out the importance of the family in current society and the strong cultural ethos regarding families (for example, anti-divorce, pro-legalized marriage) (see also Margolin, 1982). What if a therapist who is opposed to extramarital affairs begins working with a couple in which one or both partners are having affairs? Will value judgments creep into the therapy? Will the therapist view the affairs as more causal of the couple's relationship problems than might actually be the case (similar to Jamal's reaction to a client's obesity, at the beginning of this chapter)? What if a pro-choice therapist begins working with a client who turns out to be vehemently pro-life (as well as differing from the therapist on many values) and whose presenting problem involves fears of rejection and abandonment? Does the therapist work with someone whose values are nearly opposite to her or his own? Or does the therapist refer the client elsewhere and thus risk exacerbating the client's feelings of rejection and abandonment? Again, both positions can be defended on ethical grounds.

Never Stop Learning (Number 4)

Although therapists are required to stay up with current developments in the profession (like learning about the relatively new field of close relationships) and also are mandated to work only within their areas of competence, professional development does not always get the attention it merits. Many states have developed continuing education (CE) requirements for professionals licensed or certified in various mental health fields. These CE requirements facilitate professional development activities for many therapists. Just as it sometimes takes a health scare and a physician's stern warning to prompt people to take care of themselves physically, mandated CE experiences may coerce therapists to take care of themselves professionally.

Although professional growth and development is extremely important, so also is the therapist's personal life and close relationships.

The Therapist's Relationships

Several years ago, Carl Rogers defined "positive therapeutic change" as "greater integration, less internal conflict, more energy utilizable for effective living; change in behavior away from behaviors generally regarded as immature and toward behaviors regarded as mature" (1992, p. 827). Therapists could probably wish no more for themselves than what Rogers articulated as psychotherapeutic or positive personality change, and a major source of support for positive growth and change comes from the therapist's close relationships.

Although the focus in this book has been on partnered relationships, all of a therapist's close relationships are important, whether with romantic partners, children, parents, other family members, friends, or professional colleagues. And they need to be nurtured. If therapists want greater personality integration, more energy, and less conflict, then they must balance professional commitments with personal attachments in ways that maximize the quality of life.

Balance is uniquely individual, however, and it is likely that every therapist would include a somewhat different mixture of professional activities, family relationships, friends, and recreational (including exercise) activities in her or his "ideal life." In addition, activities of daily living such as eating, sleeping, household maintenance, and so on also necessitate commitments of time and energy. However, because the concept of a "relationship" may be somewhat intangible, it can be easy to defer or even ignore relationship needs and the needs of loved ones. After all, there is no state board requiring x number of units of "intimate relating" before a therapist can renew a professional license or certificate. Therapists need to care for themselves as compassionately as they do for their clients, and part of such caring involves intimate relating.

Therapist self-caring may also be accomplished through continuing or periodic experiences in supervision or therapy. Supervision can ease the awesome load of responsibility that therapists carry, and therapy can provide a forum for working out the therapist's own conflicts in a setting in which they are the receiver, rather than the giver, of nurturing. In taking care of themselves and their close relationships, therapists increase the probability that they will successfully foster growth in clients and their relationships.

In dealing with ethical and professional issues of relevance to therapists, it is interesting to consider how partners might relate differently to one another if they employed the general ethical guidelines for therapists outlined earlier in this chapter.

The Ethics of Coupling

What if romantic partners, before marrying, living together, or in any similar way formalizing their relationship, had to subscribe to an ethical code, modeled (loosely) on the AAMFT Code of Ethics? Such a Close Relationship Code of Ethics might appear this way.

I. *Responsibility to Partners*: "Persons in a romantic relationship (hereafter known as 'persons') advance the welfare of their partners."

They respect their partner's rights and make reasonable efforts to ensure that they interact with their partner appropriately. Persons don't engage in relationships that will put their partners in difficult positions. They do not use sexual involvement with the partner to substitute for emotional involvement. Persons do not prosper at their partner's expense. Persons aid partners in decision making when so invited, but the power and the responsibility are the partner's. If persons cannot be helpful to partners in a particular situation, they encourage the partner to seek help elsewhere. Finally, persons do not accept their partner's disclosure and then use it as a weapon in subsequent discussions.

II. *Confidentiality*: "Persons guard the confidentiality of their partners."

Persons break a partner's confidentiality only as required by some legal matter, when the partner represents a danger to self or others, or in some other very serious situation. In addition, persons do not gossip about their partners to other people, seeking sympathy or support for their own point of view. They work out problems with the partner directly. Not only the confidentiality of the partner but also the confidentiality of the relationship is protected.

III. *Relational Competence and Integrity*: "Persons maintain high standards of relational competence and integrity."

Persons violate the general ethical code if they break the law or engage in behavior that could lead to breaking the law. Persons also do not try to relate to their partner while impaired due to substance abuse. Persons try to get help for their problems, try to learn more about positive ways to conduct relationships, and are careful to say only what they mean, insofar as that is possible. In addition, persons try to behave ethically in all areas of their life, not just in their close relationship.

IV. *Responsibility to Others*: "Persons do not exploit other people."

Just as with their partners, persons do not exploit other people, do not get sexually involved with other people, and try not to get put in difficult relationships with other people. Persons do not betray other people's trust or confidences except as required by some legal matter, when the other people represent a danger to self or others, or in some other serious situation. Persons also conduct themselves ethically in their work/business settings and behave noncoercively.

V. *Responsibility to the Human Community*: "Persons respect other people's relationships and participate in activities that advance the goals of healthy close relationships."

Essentially, persons behave responsibly and progressively in supporting the general welfare of relationships (for example, supporting personal growth or therapy experiences for relationship partners) and promote the welfare of relationships through community involvement, relationship-supportive legislation, and so on.

VI. *Financial Arrangements*: "Persons are fair and open with their partners about all financial issues."

Persons do not encumber their partners with debts and disclose all current debts and assets. Persons are willing to share financial resources and obligations with their partners, based on agreed-upon arrangements. Persons try not to either use money as a substitute for affection or use it as an agent of aggression in the relationship. Persons are also honest in their financial dealings outside of the relationship.

VIII. *Communication and Appearance*: "Persons represent themselves honestly to potential partners and actual partners, allowing partners to make relationship choices on an informed basis."

This item refers essentially to "truth in advertising," and refers to the verbal and nonverbal behavior as well as the physical appearance that a person presents to a partner. Persons try to be as truthful as possible in what they say to their partner and to have consistent verbal and nonverbal behavior. Communication is frequent, and agreements between partners are clarified and updated as needed. Finally, things that alter the reality of appearance (for example, contact lenses, hair coloring, prostheses of any type) need to be disclosed to a partner. In addition, partners should be made aware of a person's health conditions, including HIV status.

Reading over this list of ethical concerns in close relationships, it is interesting to consider how much more difficult—and successful—relationships might be if people really adhered to rules of humanity and fairness. Because counseling couples involves the interaction of three people in an intense and intimate experience, there is an especially strong need for clear ethical and professional guidelines. The following case example illustrates some of these.

❧ *Case Example* ❧

Bill and Todd had been in a serious relationship for about four years and had lived together most of that time. Both were in their thirties. Within the past several months, their relationship had become more strained. When they were together, they fought even about little things, so each was pursuing activities with other friends and not making much time for the relationship. They realized that they were growing apart and sought relationship counseling from Allen, a marriage and family therapist who specialized in couple counseling. Allen experienced some difficulty initially in working with Bill and Todd. He had had limited experience working with gay and lesbian couples, and his own religious background included some very negative attitudes toward homosexuality. However, Bill and Todd had encountered difficulty in finding a therapist, and both seemed comfortable with Allen. Allen decided that given his general expertise in couple counseling, he needed to try to be helpful to this couple. During an individual session with Bill, he found out that Bill had begun a romantic relationship with another man, and he urged Bill to bring the affair into the open during the next couple session. The following excerpts are from halfway through the fifth session.

Therapist: I wonder if each of you could be as open and clear as possible about what changes would need to take place for you to feel satisfied with the relationship.

[Because therapist could not break client confidentiality, the therapist had to rely on the client's willingness to be honest.]

Todd: I just want to get back to the way we were. Bill is out doing things with friends nearly every night, and when he is home, I don't feel like he is really "there." We used to have a pretty active social life, and we worked out together several times a week. Now I sometimes feel like I'm living by myself.

Bill: Todd, we can't get back to the way we were. That's a lot of the problem with our relationship. You want things to stay the same, and they can't. We're not the same people we were when we first got together. I've changed jobs, you've gotten a promotion, we moved from an apartment to a house, we got a dog. We can't go back—and I don't want to. I get tired of our "social life." Everybody talks about the same things every time we get together. I'm ready to make some changes, maybe find some new friends. But every time I suggest changing anything, you get really upset and start arguing and accusing. (Both partners fall silent)

[Bill is resisting being fully honest with Todd.]

Therapist: Is that all?

Bill: No, there's something else. Todd, I have started seeing someone else. The relationship hasn't been going on very long, but . . . (Todd interrupts)

Todd: I knew there was someone else! That's what I've been afraid of, that you'd find someone else . . . and now you have. I knew you were getting tired of me.

Bill: Wait! I am getting tired of you, but not in the way you mean. And I have not found someone else. I've just gone out with this other guy a few times, and it is not sexual, believe it or not. I'm still committed to our relationship, and I still care for you very much. But you are driving me crazy. Things have got to change.

[If the outside relationship was sexual, the partners would have to deal with safe sex issues.]

Therapist: Let's just stop for a minute. Bill, you just told Todd something very important—something that he needed to know—but you need to give yourselves time to absorb it. Todd, how are you feeling right now?

Todd responds with his feelings, and Allen helps Todd and Bill begin working through the issue of Bill's involvement with someone else, believing that they will not be able to focus on their own relationship until they get at least initial resolution on the other issue. The session concludes with Allen feeling that Todd and Bill have a reasonable chance at saving their relationship.

This is Allen's last session for the evening, and on his way home he realizes that he feels sad, almost depressed. He feels good about his workday, especially that last session, so he wonders why he is feeling down. Slowly it dawns on him that in some ways he is like Bill, and his wife Stephanie is like Todd. Stephanie wants things to stay the same. She is frightened by change, and when Allen tries to change the "rules" of their relationship, she reacts with tears, or anger, or both. So he retreats into his world of work and professional colleagues. There is no "other woman," but he sometimes imagines what it would be like if there were. Then he ends up feeling guilty and trying to give Stephanie some extra attention. But tonight he thinks that maybe he will try again talking with Stephanie about his dissatisfaction with the status quo. Honest communication seemed to work for Todd and Bill; maybe it could work for him. It was both irritating and reassuring, he thought, that there's always more that you can learn about yourself, even when you are the therapist.

A number of ethical issues were involved in this case example. The therapist experienced some clash of values with his clients. He was afraid that this might negatively affect therapy, however his ethical code required him to not refuse services because of clients' sexual preference. Because he had little experience working with gay couples, he felt he might be working beyond his boundaries of competence, but the couple's issues were familiar to him. He determined that both partners were HIV-negative and were tested regularly, but if he had knowledge of a sexual affair in which one partner was practicing sexually risky behavior, the ethical issues (including confidentiality) would have become increasingly complex (see Corey et al., 1993). Although some therapists would not have promised confidentiality for information disclosed during the individual sessions, Allen felt comfortable with his approach. He relied on his clients to be honest with each other. Finally, Allen had neglected important problems in his own close relationship and realized that he needed to take some of his therapy experience and apply it to his own life. Though this last point is not part of any formal ethical code, it is of professional and personal importance to therapists.

Summary

There are a number of complex ethical and professional issues involved in counseling couples. Therapists need to understand and subscribe to the ethical guidelines relevant to their particular profession (marriage and family therapy, psychology, counseling, social work, and others). The *AAMFT Code of Ethics* (1991), for example, has sections covering responsibility to clients; confidentiality; professional competence and integrity; responsibility to students, employees, and supervisees; responsibility to research participants; responsibility to the profession; financial arrangements; and advertising. Related professional issues that occur frequently in the course of relationship counseling include determining who the client actually is, value conflicts between the therapist and clients, and the need for continued professional training and development.

Therapists also need to pay attention to and nurture their own personal relationships, understanding that the quality of their personal lives will influence the quality of their work. Finally, if partners adhered to clearly defined ethical standards in their relationships, the quality and satisfaction of intimate relationships would increase greatly.

Ultimately, we as therapists wish for ourselves what we wish for our clients: the energy, motivation, knowledge, and wisdom to nurture and enjoy the close, personal relationships that enrich our lives.

REFERENCES

ADLER, N. L., & HENDRICK, S. S. (1991). Relationships between contraceptive behavior and love attitudes, sex attitudes, and self-esteem. *Journal of Counseling and Development, 70,* 302–308.

ADLER, N. L., HENDRICK, S. S., & HENDRICK, C. (1987). Male sexual preference and attitudes toward love and sexuality. *Journal of Sex Education and Therapy, 12*(2), 27–30.

ALBRECHT, S. L., BAHR, H. M., & GOODMAN, K. L. (1983). *Divorce and remarriage: Problems, adaptations, and adjustment.* Westport, CT: Greenwood Press.

ALTMAN, I., & TAYLOR, D. A. (1973). *Social penetration: The development of interpersonal relationships.* New York: Holt, Rinehart & Winston.

AMERICAN ASSOCIATION FOR MARRIAGE AND FAMILY THERAPY. (1991). *AAMFT Code of ethics.* Washington, DC: Author.

ANDERSON, J., & WHITE, G. (1986). An empirical investigation of interactive and relationship patterns in functional and dysfunctional nuclear families and stepfamilies. *Family Process, 25,* 407–422.

ARON, A., DUTTON, D. G., ARON, E. N., & IVERSON, A. (1989). Experiences of falling in love. *Journal of Social and Personal Relationships, 6,* 243–257.

ARONSON, E., WILLERMAN, B., & FLOYD, J. (1966). The effect of a pratfall on increasing interpersonal attractiveness. *Psychonomic Science, 4,* 227–228.

BABCOCK, J. C., WALTZ, J., JACOBSON, N. S., & GOTTMAN, J. M. (1993). Power and violence: The relation between communication patterns, power discrepancies, and domestic violence. *Journal of Consulting and Clinical Psychology, 61,* 40–50.

BAILEY, W. C., HENDRICK, C., & HENDRICK, S. S. (1987). Relation of sex and gender role to love, sexual attitudes, and self-esteem. *Sex Roles, 16,* 637–648.

BARBER, B. L., & ECCLES, J. S. (1992). Long-term influence of divorce and single parenting on adolescent family- and work-related values, behaviors, and aspirations. *Psychological Bulletin, 111*, 108–126.

BARNETT, R. C., MARSHALL, N. L., & PLECK, J. H. (1992). Men's multiple roles and their relationship to men's psychological distress. *Journal of Marriage and the Family, 54*, 358–367.

BARUTH, L. G., & HUBER, C. H. (1984). *An introduction to marital theory and therapy*. Pacific Grove, CA: Brooks/Cole.

BAXTER, L. A. (1990). Dialectical contradictions in relationship development. *Journal of Social and Personal Relationships, 7*, 69–88.

BAXTER, L. A., & BULLIS, C. (1986). Turning points in developing romantic relationships. *Human Communication Research, 12*, 469–493.

BECVAR, D. S., & BECVAR, R. J. (1988). *Family therapy: A systemic integration*. Boston: Allyn & Bacon.

BELENKY, M. F., CLINCHY, B. M., GOLDBERGER, N. R., & TARULE, J. M. (1986). *Women's ways of knowing*. New York: Basic Books.

BEM, S. L. (1974). The measurement of psychological androgyny. *Journal of Consulting and Clinical Psychology, 42*, 155–162.

BENNETT, B. E., BRYANT, B. K., VANDENBOS, G. R., & GREENWOOD, A. (1990). *Professional liability and risk management*. Washington, DC: American Psychological Association.

BERARDO, D. H., SHEHAN, C. L., & LESLIE, G. R. (1987). A residue of tradition: Jobs, careers, and spouses' time in housework. *Journal of Marriage and the Family, 49*, 381–390.

BERG, J. H., & CLARK, M. S. (1986). Differences in social exchange between intimate and other relationships: Gradually evolving or quickly apparent? In V. J. Derlega & B. A. Winstead (Eds.), *Friendship and social interaction* (pp. 101–128). New York: Springer-Verlag.

BERNARD, J. (1972). *The future of marriage*. New York: World.

BERSCHEID, E., DION, K., WALSTER, E., & WALSTER, G. W. (1971). Physical attractiveness and dating choice: A test of the matching hypothesis. *Journal of Experimental Social Psychology, 1*, 173–189.

BERSCHEID, E., & WALSTER, E. (1978). *Interpersonal attraction* (2nd ed.). Reading, MA: Addison-Wesley.

BERZON, B. (1988). *Permanent partners: Building gay & lesbian relationships that last*. New York: Plume.

BLIESZNER, R., & ADAMS, R. G. (1992). *Adult friendship*. Thousand Oaks, CA: Sage.

BLOOM, B. L., ASHER, S. J., & WHITE, S. W. (1978). Marital disruption as a stressor: A review and analysis. *Psychological Bulletin, 85*, 867–894.

BLUMSTEIN, P., & SCHWARTZ, P. (1983). *American couples*. New York: William Morrow.

BOHANNAN, P. (Ed.). (1970). *Divorce and after*. Garden City, NY: Doubleday.

BOHANNAN, P. (1984). *All the happy families: Exploring the varieties of family life.* New York: McGraw-Hill.

BOWEN, M. (1978). *Family therapy in clinical practice.* New York: Aronson.

BRADBURY, T. N., & FINCHAM, F. D. (1992). Attributions and behavior in marital interaction. *Journal of Personality and Social Psychology, 63,* 613–628.

BRICKMAN, P. (1974). Rule structures and conflict relationships. In P. Brickman (Ed.), *Social conflict.* Lexington, MA: D. C. Heath.

BRODY, G. H., NEUBAUM, E., & FOREHAND, R. (1988). Serial marriage: A heuristic analysis of an emerging family form. *Psychological Bulletin, 103,* 211–222.

BROWN, M., & AUERBACK, A. (1981). Communication patterns in initiation of marital sex. *Medical Aspects of Human Sexuality, 15,* 105–117.

BURKE, P. J., STETS, J. E., & PIROG-GOOD, M. A. (1988). Gender identity, self-esteem, and physical and sexual abuse in dating relationships. *Social Psychology Quarterly, 51,* 272–285.

BURKE, R. J., WEIR, T., & HARRISON, D. (1976). Disclosure of problems and tensions experienced by marital partners. *Psychological Reports, 38,* 531–542.

BURMAN, B., & MARGOLIN, G. (1992). Analysis of the association between marital relationships and health problems: An interactional perspective. *Psychological Bulletin, 112,* 39–63.

BURR, W. R. (1973). *Theory construction and the sociology of the family.* New York: Wiley.

BUSS, D. M., & BARNES, M. (1986). Preferences in human mate selection. *Journal of Personality and Social Psychology, 50,* 559–570.

BYRNE, D. (1971). *The attraction paradigm.* New York: Academic Press.

BYRNE, D., CLORE, G. L., JR., & WORCHEL, P. (1966). Effect of economic similarity-dissimilarity on interpersonal attraction. *Journal of Personality and Social Psychology, 4,* 220–224.

CALDWELL, M. A., & PEPLAU, L. A. (1982). Sex differences in same-sex friendship. *Sex Roles, 8,* 721–732.

CATE, R. M., HUSTON, T. L., & NESSELROADE, J. R. (1986). Premarital relationships: Toward the identification of alternative pathways to marriage. *Journal of Social and Clinical Psychology, 4,* 3–22.

CATE, R. M., & LLOYD, S. A. (1988). Courtship. In S. Duck (Ed.), *Handbook of personal relationships: Theory, research and interventions* (pp. 409–427). New York: Wiley.

CHRISTOPHER, F. S., & CATE, R. M. (1984). Factors involved in premarital sexual decision-making. *The Journal of Sex Research, 20,* 363–376.

CHRISTOPHER, F. S., & FRANDSEN, M. M. (1990). Strategies of influence in sex and dating. *Journal of Social and Personal Relationships, 7,* 89–105.

COBB, S. (1976). Social support as a moderator of life stress. *Psychosomatic Medicine, 38,* 300–314.

COLEMAN, M., & GANONG, L. H. (1990). Remarriage and stepfamily research in the 1980s: Increased interest in an old family form. *Journal of Marriage and the Family, 52,* 925–940.

CONSTANTINE, L. L. (1986). Jealousy and extramarital sexual relations. In N. S. Jacobson & A. S. Gurman (Eds.), *Clinical handbook of marital therapy* (pp. 407–427). New York: Guilford.

CONTRERAS, R., HENDRICK, S. S., & HENDRICK, C. (1994). Perspectives on marital love and satisfaction in Mexican American and Anglo couples. Manuscript under review.

COREY, G., COREY, M. S., & CALLANAN, P. (1993). *Issues and ethics in the helping professions.* Pacific Grove, CA: Brooks/Cole.

CUPACH, W. R. (1992). Dialectical processes in the disengagement of interpersonal relationships. In T. L. Orbuch (Ed.), *Close relationship loss: Theoretical approaches* (pp. 128–141). New York: Springer-Verlag.

CUPACH, W. R., & COMSTOCK, J. (1990). Satisfaction with sexual communication in marriage: Links to sexual satisfaction and dyadic adjustment. *Journal of Social and Personal Relationships, 7,* 179–186.

CURRAN, J. P. (1975). Convergence toward a single sexual standard? *Social Behavior and Personality, 3,* 189–195.

CUTRONA, C. E., SUHR, J. A., & MACFARLANE, R. (1990). Interpersonal transactions and the psychological sense of support. In S. Duck & R. Silver (Eds.), *Personal relationships and social support* (pp. 30–45). London: Sage.

CUTRONA, C. E., & SUHR, J. A. (1994). Social support communication in the context of marriage: An analysis of couples' supportive interactions. In B. R. Burleson, T. L. Albrecht, & I. G. Sarason (Eds.), *Communication of social support: Messages, interactions, relationships, and community* (pp. 113–135). Thousand Oaks, CA: Sage.

DARE, C. (1986). Psychoanalytic marital therapy. In N. S. Jacobson & A. S. Gurman (Eds.), *Clinical handbook of marital therapy* (pp. 13–28). New York: Guilford.

DATTILIO, F. M., & PADESKY, C. A. (1990). *Cognitive therapy with couples.* Sarasota, FL: Professional Resource Exchange.

DAVIS, K. E., & TODD, M. (1982). Friendship and love relationships. In K. E. Davis (Ed.), *Advances in descriptive psychology* (Vol. 2, pp. 79–122). Greenwich, CT: JAI Press.

DEAUX, K. (1993). Commentary: Sorry, wrong number—a reply to Gentile's call. *Psychological Science, 4,* 125–126.

DEMARIS, A., & RAO, K. V. (1992). Premarital cohabitation and subsequent marital stability in the United States: A reassessment. *Journal of Marriage and the Family, 54,* 178–190.

DERLEGA, V. J., HENDRICK, S. S., WINSTEAD, B. A., & BERG, J. H. (1991). *Psychotherapy as a personal relationship.* New York: Guilford.

DERLEGA, V. J., METTS, S., PETRONIO, S., & MARGULIS, S. T. (1993). *Self-disclosure.* Thousand Oaks, CA: Sage.

DERLEGA, V. J., WINSTEAD, B. A., WONG, P. T. P., & HUNTER, S. (1985). Gender effects in an initial encounter: A case where men exceed women in disclosure. *Journal of Social and Personal Relationships, 2,* 25–44.

DINDIA, K., & ALLEN, M. (1992). Sex differences in self-disclosure: A meta-analysis. *Psychological Bulletin, 112,* 106–124.

DOWNEY, D. B., & POWELL, B. (1993). Do children in single-parent households fare better living with same-sex parents? *Journal of Marriage and the Family, 55,* 55–71.

DRIGOTAS, S. M., & RUSBULT, C. E. (1992). Should I stay or should I go? A dependence model of breakups. *Journal of Personality and Social Psychology, 62,* 62–87.

DUCK, S. (1982). A topography of relationship disengagement and dissolution. In S. Duck (Ed.), *Personal relationships 4: Dissolving personal relationships* (pp. 1–30). New York: Academic Press.

DUCK, S., & SANTS, H. (1983). On the origin of the specious: Are personal relationships really interpersonal states? *Journal of Social and Clinical Psychology, 1,* 27–41.

ELDRIDGE, N. S., & GILBERT, L. A. (1990). Correlates of relationship satisfaction in lesbian couples. *Psychology of Women Quarterly, 14,* 43–62.

FALBO, T., & PEPLAU, L. A. (1980). Power strategies in intimate relationships. *Journal of Personality and Social Psychology, 38,* 618–628.

FEHR, B. (1988). Prototype analysis of the concepts of love and commitment. *Journal of Personality and Social Psychology, 55,* 557–579.

FEINGOLD, A. (1988). Matching for attractiveness in romantic partners and same-sex friends: A meta-analysis and theoretical critique. *Psychological Bulletin, 104,* 226–235.

FINE, M. A., & FINE, D. R. (1992). Recent changes in laws affecting stepfamilies: Suggestions for legal reform. *Family Relations, 41,* 334–340.

FITZPATRICK, M. A. (1988a). Approaches to marital interaction. In P. Noller & M. A. Fitzpatrick (Eds.), *Perspectives on marital interaction* (pp. 1–28). Philadelphia: Multilingual Matters.

FITZPATRICK, M. A. (1988b). A typological approach to marital interaction. In P. Noller & M. A. Fitzpatrick (Eds.), *Perspectives on marital interaction* (pp. 98–120). Philadelphia: Multilingual Matters.

FOSTER, S. W. (1986). Marital treatment of eating disorders. In N. S. Jacobson & A. S. Gurman (Eds.), *Clinical handbook of marital therapy* (pp. 575–593). New York: Guilford.

FRAZIER, P. A., & COOK, S. W. (1993). Correlates of distress following heterosexual relationship dissolution. *Journal of Social and Personal Relationships, 10,* 55–67.

FRENCH, J. R. P., & RAVEN, B. (1968). The bases of social power. In D. Cartwright & A. Zander (Eds.), *Group dynamics: Research and theory* (3rd ed.) (pp. 259–269). New York: Harper & Row.

FRIEZE, I. H., & MCHUGH, M. C. (1992). Power and influence strategies in violent and nonviolent marriages. *Psychology of Women Quarterly, 16,* 449–465.

FURSTENBERG, F. F. (1987). The new extended family: The experience of parents and children after remarriage. In K. Pasley & M. Ihinger-Tallman (Eds.), *Remarriage and stepparenting: Current research and theory* (pp. 42–61). New York: Guilford.

GAELICK, L., BODENHAUSEN, G. V., & WYER, R. S., JR. (1985). Emotional communication in close relationships. *Journal of Personality and Social Psychology, 49,* 1246–1265.

GELLES, R. J., & CORNELL, C. P. (1985). *Intimate violence in families.* Thousand Oaks, CA: Sage.

GENTILE, D. A. (1993). Just what are sex and gender, anyway? A call for a new terminological standard. *Psychological Science, 4,* 120–122.

GILBERT, L. A. (1988). *Sharing it all: The rewards and struggles of two-career families.* New York: Plenum.

GILBERT, L. A. (1993). *Two careers/one family: The promise of gender equality.* Thousand Oaks, CA: Sage.

GILLIGAN, C. (1982). *In a different voice.* Cambridge, MA: Harvard University Press.

GLENN, N. D. (1990). Quantitative research on marital quality in the 1980s: A critical review. *Journal of Marriage and the Family, 52,* 818–831.

GOLDBERG, D. C., (Ed.). (1985). *Contemporary marriage: Special issues in couples therapy.* Pacific Grove, CA: Brooks/Cole.

GOLDENBERG, H., & GOLDENBERG, I. (1990). *Counseling today's families.* Pacific Grove, CA: Brooks/Cole.

GREEN, S. L., & HANSEN, J. C. (1989). Ethical dilemmas faced by family therapists. *Journal of Marital and Family Therapy, 15,* 149–158.

HALEY, J. (1987). *Problem-solving therapy* (2nd ed.). San Francisco: Jossey-Bass.

HATFIELD, E., & SPRECHER, S. (1986). Measuring passionate love in intimate relations. *Journal of Adolescence, 9,* 383–410.

HAZAN, C., & SHAVER, P. (1987). Romantic love conceptualized as an attachment process. *Journal of Personality and Social Psychology, 52,* 511–524.

HENDRICK, C., & HENDRICK, S. S. (1986). A theory and method of love. *Journal of Personality and Social Psychology, 50,* 392–402.

HENDRICK, C., & HENDRICK, S. S. (1988). Lovers wear rose colored glasses. *Journal of Social and Personal Relationships, 5,* 161–183.

HENDRICK, S. S. (1981). Self-disclosure and marital satisfaction. *Journal of Personality and Social Psychology, 40,* 1150–1159.

HENDRICK, S. S. (1988). A generic measure of relationship satisfaction. *Journal of Marriage and the Family, 50,* 93–98.

HENDRICK, S. S., & HENDRICK, C. (1987). Love and sexual attitudes, self-disclosure and sensation seeking. *Journal of Social and Personal Relationships, 4,* 281–297.

HENDRICK, S. S., & HENDRICK, C. (1992a). *Liking, loving, & relating* (2nd ed.). Pacific Grove, CA: Brooks/Cole.

HENDRICK, S. S., & HENDRICK, C. (1992b). *Romantic love.* Thousand Oaks, CA: Sage.

HENDRICK, S. S., & HENDRICK, C. (1993). Lovers as friends. *Journal of Social and Personal Relationships, 10,* 459–466.

HENDRICK, S. S., HENDRICK, C., & ADLER, N. L. (1988). Romantic relationships: Love, satisfaction, and staying together. *Journal of Personality and Social Psychology, 54,* 980–988.

HETHERINGTON, E. M. (1987). Family relations six years after divorce. In K. Pasley & M. Ihinger-Tallman (Eds.), *Remarriage and stepparenting: Current research and theory* (pp. 185–205). New York: Guilford.

HILL, C. T., & STULL, D. E. (1987). Gender and self-disclosure: Strategies for exploring the issues. In V. J. Derlega & J. H. Berg (Eds.), *Self-disclosure: Theory, research and therapy* (pp. 81–100). New York: Plenum.

HOCHSCHILD, A. R. (1989). *The second shift: Working parents and the revolution at home.* New York: Viking.

HOLMES, J. G., & REMPEL, J. K. (1989). Trust in close relationships. In C. Hendrick (Ed.), *Close relationships* (pp. 187–220). Thousand Oaks, CA: Sage.

HOWARD, J. A., BLUMSTEIN, P., & SCHWARTZ, P. (1986). Sex, power, and influence tactics in intimate relationships. *Journal of Personality and Social Psychology, 51,* 102–109.

HUSTON, T. L., & VANGELISTI, A. L. (1991). Socioemotional behavior and satisfaction in marital relationships: A longitudinal study. *Journal of Personality and Social Psychology, 61,* 721–733.

JACOBS, J. E., & ECCLES, J. S. (1992). The impact of mothers' gender-role stereotypic beliefs on mothers' and children's ability perceptions. *Journal of Personality and Social Psychology, 63,* 932–944.

JACOBSON, N. S., & GURMAN, A. S. (Eds.). (1986). *Clinical handbook of marital therapy.* New York: Guilford.

JACOBSON, N. S., & HOLTZWORTH-MUNROE, A. (1986). Marital therapy: A social learning-cognitive perspective. In N. S. Jacobson & A. S.

Gurman (Eds.), *Clinical handbook of marital therapy* (pp. 29–70). New York: Guilford.

JACOBSON, N. S., MCDONALD, D. W., FOLLETTE, W. C., & BERLEY, R. A. (1985). Attributional processes in distressed and nondistressed married couples. *Cognitive Therapy and Research, 9*, 35–50.

JAMES, W. H. (1981). The honeymoon effect on marital coitus. *The Journal of Sex Research, 17*, 114–123.

JORGENSEN, S. R., & GAUDY, J. C. (1980). Self-disclosure and satisfaction in marriage: The relation examined. *Family Relations, 29*, 281–287.

JOURARD, S. M. (1964). *The transparent self.* Princeton, NJ: Van Nostrand Reinhold.

KASLOW, F. W., & SCHWARTZ, L. L. (1987). *The dynamics of divorce: A life cycle perspective.* New York: Brunner/Mazel.

KEITH-SPIEGEL, P., & KOOCHER, G. (1985). *Ethics in psychology: Professional standards and cases.* New York: Random House.

KITSON, G. C., & MORGAN, L. A. (1990). The multiple consequences of divorce: A decade review. *Journal of Marriage and the Family, 52*, 913–924.

KLEINKE, C. L. (1986). Gaze and eye contact: A research review. *Psychological Bulletin, 100*, 78–100.

KOSS, M. P. (1988). Hidden rape: Incidence, prevalence, and descriptive characteristics of sexual aggression and victimization in a national sample of college students. In W. A. Burgess (Ed.), *Sexual assault: Vol. II* (pp. 1–25). New York: Garland.

KURDEK, L. A. (1991). The relations between reported well-being and divorce history, availability of a proximate adult, and gender. *Journal of Marriage and the Family, 53*, 71–78.

KURDEK, L. A. (1992). Relationship stability and relationship satisfaction in cohabiting gay and lesbian couples: A prospective longitudinal test of the contextual and interdependence models. *Journal of Social and Personal Relationships, 9*, 125–142.

KURDEK, L. A., & SCHMITT, J. P. (1986). Early development of relationship quality in heterosexual married, heterosexual cohabiting, gay, and lesbian couples. *Developmental Psychology, 22*, 305–309.

LASSWELL, M., & LOBSENZ, N. M. (1980). *Styles of loving: Why you love the way you do.* New York: Doubleday.

LEE, J. A. (1973). *The colors of love: An exploration of the ways of loving.* Don Mills, Ontario: New Press.

LEVINGER, G. (1979). Marital cohesiveness at the brink: The fate of applications for divorce. In G. Levinger & O. C. Moles (Eds.), *Divorce and separation.* New York: Basic Books.

LEVINGER, G., & SENN, D. J. (1967). Disclosure of feelings in marriage. *Merrill-Palmer Quarterly, 13*, 237–249.

LLOYD, K., PAULSEN, J., & BROCKNER, J. (1983). The effects of self-esteem and self-consciousness on interpersonal attraction. *Personality and Social Psychology Bulletin, 9*, 397–403.

LLOYD, S. A., & CATE, R. M. (1985). The developmental course of conflict in dissolution of premarital relationships. *Journal of Social and Personal Relationships, 2*, 179–194.

LOWERY, C. R., & SETTLE, S. A. (1985). Effects of divorce on children: Differential impact of custody and visitation patterns. *Family Relations, 34*, 455–463.

LUKAS, S. (1993). *Where to start and what to ask: An assessment handbook.* New York: Norton.

MARGOLIN, G. (1982). Ethical and legal considerations in marital and family therapy. *American Psychologist, 37*, 788–801.

MCHALE, S. M., & CROUTER, A. C. (1992). You can't always get what you want: Incongruence between sex–role attitudes and family work roles and its implications for marriage. *Journal of Marriage and the Family, 54*, 537–547.

MENAGHAN, E. G., & PARCEL, T. L. (1990). Parental employment and family life: Research in the 1980s. *Journal of Marriage and the Family, 52*, 1079–1098.

MILLER, L. C., BERG, J. H., & ARCHER, R. L. (1983). Openers: Individuals who elicit intimate self-disclosure. *Journal of Personality and Social Psychology, 44*, 1234–1244.

MINUCHIN, S. (1974). *Families & family therapy.* Cambridge, MA: Harvard University Press.

MINUCHIN, S., & NICHOLS, M. P. (1993). *Family healing: Tales of hope and renewal from family therapy.* New York: The Free Press.

MORIN, S. F. (1977). Heterosexual bias in psychological research on lesbianism and male homosexuality. *American Psychologist, 32*, 629–637.

MUEHLENHARD, C. L. (1988). Misinterpreted dating behaviors and the risk of date rape. *Journal of Social and Clinical Psychology, 6*, 20–37.

MUEHLENHARD, C. L., & HOLLABAUGH, L. S. (1988). Do women sometimes say no when they mean yes? The prevalence and correlates of women's token resistance to sex. *Journal of Personality and Social Psychology, 54*, 872–879.

MURSTEIN, B. I. (1976). *Who will marry whom?* New York: Springer.

MURSTEIN, B. I., & CHRISTY, P. (1976). Physical attractivensss and marriage adjustment in middle-aged couples. *Journal of Personality and Social Psychology, 34*, 537–542.

MYERS, I. B., & MCCAULLEY, M. H. (1985). *Manual: A guide to the development and use of the Myers-Briggs Type Indicator.* Palo Alto, CA: Consulting Psychologists Press.

NEVID, J. S. (1984). Sex differences in factors of romantic attraction. *Sex Roles, 11*, 401–411.

NEWCOMB, M. D. (1986). Cohabitation, marriage and divorce among adolescents and young adults. *Journal of Social and Personal Relationships, 3*, 473—494.

NOLLER, P., & VENARDOS, C. (1986). Communication awareness in married couples. *Journal of Social and Personal Relationships, 3*, 31—42.

O'FARRELL, T. J. (1986). Marital therapy in the treatment of alcoholism. In N. S. Jacobson & A. S. Gurman (Eds.), *Clinical handbook of marital therapy* (pp. 513–535). New York: Guilford.

ORLINSKY, D. E., & HOWARD, K. I. (1986). Process and outcome in psychotherapy. In S. L. Garfield & A. E. Bergin (Eds.), *Handbook of psychotherapy and behavior change* (3rd ed.) (pp. 311–381). New York: Wiley.

ORVIS, B. R., KELLEY, H. H., & BUTLER, D. (1976). Attributional conflict in young couples. In J. H. Harvey, W. J. Ickes, & R. F. Kidd (Eds.), *New directions in attribution research* (Vol. 1, pp. 353–386). Hillsdale, NJ: Erlbaum.

PENNEBAKER, J. W. (1990). *Opening up: The healing power of confiding in others.* New York: Morrow.

PEPLAU, L. A., RUBIN, Z., & HILL, C. T. (1977). Sexual intimacy in dating relationships. *Journal of Social Issues, 33*(2), 86–109.

PETERSON, D. R. (1983). Conflict. In H. H. Kelley, E. Berscheid, A. Christensen, J. H. Harvey, T. L. Huston, G. Levinger, E. McClintock, L. A. Peplau, & D. R. Peterson (Eds.), *Close relationships* (pp. 360–396). New York: W. H. Freeman.

PETERSON, R. R. (1989). *Women, work, and divorce.* Albany, NY: SUNY Press.

PIERCE, G. R., SARASON, B. R., & SARASON, I. G. (1992). General and specific support expectations and stress as predictors of perceived supportiveness: An experimental study. *Journal of Personality and Social Psychology, 63*, 297–307.

PIERCE, G. R., SARASON, I. G., & SARASON, B. R. (1991). General and relationship-based perceptions of social support: Are two constructs better than one? *Journal of Personality and Social Psychology, 61*, 1028–1039.

PLECK, J. H. (1985). *Working wives/working husbands.* Thousand Oaks, CA: Sage.

POPE, K. S., & VASQUEZ, M. J. T. (1991). *Ethics in psychotherapy and counseling: A practical guide for psychologists.* San Francisco: Jossey-Bass.

PRINS, K. S., BUUNK, B. P., & VANYPEREN, N. W. (1993). Equity, normative disapproval and extramarital relationships. *Journal of Social and Personal Relationships, 10,* 39–53.

RACHLIN, V. C. (1987). Fair vs. equal role relations in dual-career and dual-earner families: Implications for family interventions. *Family Relations, 36,* 187–192.

RAINS, P. M. (1971). *Becoming an unwed mother.* Chicago: Aldine.

REISS, I. L., BANWART, A., & FOREMAN, H. (1975). Premarital contraceptive usage: A study and some theoretical explorations. *Journal of Marriage and the Family, 37,* 619–630.

REISS, I. L., & LEE, G. R. (1988). *Family systems in America* (4th ed.). New York: Holt, Rinehart & Winston.

RICHARDSON, D. R., MEDVIN, N., & HAMMOCK, G. (1988). Love styles, relationship experience, and sensation seeking: A test of validity. *Personality and Individual Differences, 9,* 645–651.

ROGERS, C. R. (1992). The necessary and sufficient conditions of therapeutic personality change. *Journal of Consulting and Clinical Psychology, 60,* 827–832. (Reprinted from *Journal of Consulting Psychology, 21,* 95–103.)

ROLLINS, B., & CANNON, K. (1974). Marital satisfaction over the family life cycle: A reevaluation. *Journal of Marriage and the Family, 36,* 271–282.

ROSENBAUM, A., & O'LEARY, K. D. (1986). The treatment of marital violence. In N. S. Jacobson & A. S. Gurman (Eds.), *Clinical handbook of marital therapy* (pp. 385–405). New York: Guilford.

RUBIN, Z. (1970). Measurement of romantic love. *Journal of Personality and Social Psychology, 16,* 265–273.

RUBIN, Z. (1973). *Liking and loving: An invitation to social psychology.* New York: Holt, Rinehart & Winston.

RUSBULT, C. E. (1983). A longitudinal test of the investment model: The development (and deterioration) of satisfaction and commitment in heterosexual involvements. *Journal of Personality and Social Psychology, 45,* 101–117.

RUSBULT, C. E., JOHNSON, D. J., & MORROW, G. D. (1986). Impact of couple patterns of problem solving on distress and nondistress in dating relationships. *Journal of Personality and Social Psychology, 50,* 744–753.

SAFRAN, J. D., & SEGAL, Z. V. (1990). *Interpersonal process in cognitive therapy.* New York: Basic Books.

SAGRESTANO, L. M. (1992). Power strategies in interpersonal relationships: The effects of expertise and gender. *Psychology of Women Quarterly, 16,* 481–495.

SANTROCK, J. W., & SITTERLE, K. A. (1987). Parent-child relationships in stepmother families. In K. Pasley & M. Ihinger-Tallman (Eds.), *Remarriage and stepparenting: Current research and theory* (pp. 273–299). New York: Guilford.

SATIR, V. (1967). *Conjoint family therapy.* Palo Alto, CA: Science and Behavior Books.

SATIR, V., & BALDWIN, M. (1983). *Satir step by step: A guide to creating change in families.* Palo Alto, CA: Science and Behavior Books.

SCANZONI, J., POLONKO, K., TEACHMAN, J., & THOMPSON, L. (1989). *The sexual bond: Rethinking families and close relationships.* Thousand Oaks, CA: Sage.

SELVINI PALAZZOLI, M., BOSCOLO, L., CECCHIN, G., & PRATA, G. (1978). *Paradox and counterparadox.* New York: Aronson.

SEYFRIED, B. A., & HENDRICK, C. (1973). When do opposites attract? When they are opposite in sex and sex-role attitudes. *Journal of Personality and Social Psychology, 25,* 15–20.

SHERROD, D. (1989). The influence of gender on same-sex friendships. In C. Hendrick (Ed.), *Close relationships* (pp. 164–186). Thousand Oaks, CA: Sage.

SHOTLAND, R. L. (1989). A model of the causes of date rape in developing and close relationships. In C. Hendrick (Ed.), *Close relationships* (pp. 247–270). Thousand Oaks, CA: Sage.

SIMPSON, J. A., CAMPBELL, B., & BERSCHEID, E. (1986). The association between romantic love and marriage: Kephart (1967) twice revisited. *Personality and Social Psychology Bulletin, 12,* 363–372.

SMITH, T. A. (1992). Family cohesion in remarried families. *Journal of Divorce & Remarriage, 17*(1/2), 49–66.

SNYDER, D. K. (1979). *Marital Satisfaction Inventory.* Los Angeles: Western Psychological Services.

SPANIER, G. B. (1976). Measuring dyadic adjustment: New scales for assessing the quality of marriage and similar dyads. *Journal of Marriage and the Family, 38,* 15–25.

SPRECHER, S. (1991). The impact of the threat of AIDS on heterosexual dating relationships. *Journal of Psychology and Human Sexuality, 3,* 3–23.

SPRECHER, S., & MCKINNEY, K. (1993). *Sexuality.* Thousand Oaks, CA: Sage.

SPRECHER, S., MCKINNEY, K., & ORBUCH, T. L. (1987). Has the double standard disappeared? An experimental test. *Social Psychology Quarterly, 50,* 24–31.

STEIL, J. M., & WELTMAN, K. (1992). Influence strategies at home and at work: A study of sixty dual career couples. *Journal of Social and Personal Relationships, 9,* 65–88.

STERNBERG, R. J. (1986). A triangular theory of love. *Psychological Review, 93*, 119–135.

STERNBERG, R. J. (1987). Liking versus loving: A comparative evaluation of theories. *Psychological Bulletin, 102*, 331–345.

STRAUS, M. A., & GELLES, R. J. (1990). *Physical violence in American families*. New Brunswick, NJ: Transaction Publishers.

STUART, R. B. (1980). *Helping couples change: A social learning approach to marital therapy*. New York: Guilford.

SURRA, C. A. (1987). Reasons for changes in commitment: Variations by courtship type. *Journal of Social and Personal Relationships, 4*, 17–33.

SURRA, C. A. (1990). Research and theory on mate selection and premarital relationships in the 1980s. *Journal of Marriage and the Family, 52*, 844–865.

TAVRIS, C. (1992). *The mismeasure of woman*. New York: Simon & Schuster.

THOMAS, S., ALBRECHT, K., & WHITE, P. (1984). Determinants of marital quality in dual-career couples. *Family Relations, 33*, 513–521.

THOMSON, E., & COLELLA, U. (1992). Cohabitation and marital stability: Quality or commitment. *Journal of Marriage and the Family, 54*, 259–267.

TODD, T. C. (1986). Structural-strategic marital therapy. In N. S. Jacobson & A. S. Gurman (Eds.), *Clinical handbook of marital therapy* (pp. 71–105). New York: Guilford.

TUCKER, M. B., & MITCHELL-KERNAN, C. (1990). New trends in black American interracial marriage: The social structural context. *Journal of Marriage and the Family, 52*, 209–218.

VANNOY, D., & PHILLIBER, W. W. (1992). Wife's employment and quality of marriage. *Journal of Marriage and the Family, 54*, 387–398.

VISHER, E. B., & VISHER, J. S. (1979). *Stepfamilies: A guide to working with stepparents and stepchildren*. New York: Brunner/Mazel.

VISHER, E. B., & VISHER, J. S. (1988). *Old loyalties, new ties: Therapeutic strategies with stepfamilies*. New York: Brunner/Mazel.

WALSH, W. M. (1992). Twenty major issues in remarriage families. *Journal of Counseling & Development, 70*, 709–715.

WALSTER, E., BERSCHEID, E., & WALSTER, G. W. (1973). New directions in equity research. *Journal of Personality and Social Psychology, 25*, 151–176.

WALSTER, E., BERSCHEID, E., & WALSTER, G. W. (1976). New directions in equity research. In L. Berkowitz & E. Walster (Eds.), *Advances in experimental social psychology: Equity theory: Toward a general theory of social interaction* (Vol. 9) (pp. 1–42). New York: Academic Press.

WALSTER, E., & WALSTER, G. W. (1978). *A new look at love*. Reading, MA: Addison-Wesley.

WALTERS, M., CARTER, B., PAPP, P., & SILVERSTEIN, O. (1988). *The invisible web: Gender patterns in family relationships*. New York: Guilford.

WEARY, G., STANLEY, M. A., & HARVEY, J. H. (1989). *Attribution*. New York: Springer-Verlag.

WEISHAUS, S., & FIELD, D. (1988). A half century of marriage: Continuity or change? *Journal of Marriage and the Family, 50,* 763–774.

WILLS, T. A., WEISS, R. I, & PATTERSON, G. R. (1974). A behavioral analysis of the determinants of marital satisfaction. *Journal of Consulting and Clinical Psychology, 42,* 802–811.

WINCH, R. F. (1958). *Mate selection: A study of complementary needs*. New York: Harper & Brothers.

WORDEN, M. (1994). *Family therapy basics*. Pacific Grove, CA: Brooks/Cole.

WORTMAN, C. B., & DUNKEL-SCHETTER, C. (1987). Conceptual and methodological issues in the study of social support. In A. Baum & J. E. Singer (Eds.), *Handbook of psychology and health, Vol. 5: Stress* (pp. 63–108). Hillsdale, NJ: Erlbaum.

ZUO, J. (1992). The reciprocal relationship between marital interaction and marital happiness: A three-wave study. *Journal of Marriage and the Family, 54,* 870–878.

INDEX

AAMFT. *See* American Association for Marriage and Family Therapy
Abuse
  spouse, 11–12, 80–81
  substance, 11, 94
Adams, R. G., 68
Adjustment, in close relationships, 58–60
Adler, N. L., 31, 41, 61
Adult recovery, divorce and, 100
Advertising, therapist ethics and, 114–115
Affairs, extramarital. *See* Infidelity
Affection, relational satisfaction and, 40
Agape, as love style, 26, 29, 30
AIDS
  infidelity and, 11
  sexual self-disclosure and, 41, 120, 123
Albrecht, K., 83
Albrecht, S. L., 94
Alcoholics Anonymous (AA), 11
Alcoholism, 11, 98
Allen, M., 45
Altman, I., 44
American Association for Marriage and Family Therapy (AAMFT), code of ethics of, 112–115, 118, 123
Anderson, J., 102
Archer, R. L., 50
Aron, A., 21
Aron, E. N., 21
Aronson, E., 20
Asher, S. J., 98
Assessment, in couple counseling, 10–12
Attraction

factors in, 18–21
sexual, 38–40
Attractiveness. *See* Physical attractiveness
Attributions, conflict and, 64–65
Auerback, A., 47
Autonomy-connection contradiction, 47, 92
Avoiders, 63

Babcock, J. C., 63, 80
Bahr, H. M., 94
Bailey, W. C., 30
Baldwin, M., 14, 15
Banwart, A., 41
Barber, B. L., 99
Barnes, M., 38
Barnett, R. C., 83
Baruth, L. G., 4, 12, 13
Baxter, L. A., 39, 47
Becvar, D. S., 15
Becvar, R. J., 15
Behavior
  couple counseling and, 13–14
  task vs. emotional, 61
Belenky, M. F., 76
Bem Sex Role Inventory, 30
Bem, S. L., 30
Bennett, B. E., 112
Berardo, D. H., 84
Berg, J. H., 5, 44, 50
Berley, R. A., 65
Bernard, J., 60
Berscheid, E., 20, 22, 24
Berzon, B., 40, 61, 68, 85
Biological-discrimination hypothesis, 102

Compatibility, 21
Competence
    relational, 119
    therapist ethics and, 113
Complementarity, 18, 21
Compromise stage, of conflict, 62
Comstock, J., 48
Confidentiality
    in close relationships, 119
    therapist ethics and, 113
Conflict
    attributions and, 64–65
    in close relationships, 62–63
Constantine, L. L., 11
Continuing education, for thera-
        pists, 117
Contraceptive behavior, 41
Contradictions, in close relationships,
        47, 92–93
Contreras, R., 29, 31, 58
Cook, S. W., 100
Coparental divorce, 96
Corey, G., 112, 115, 116, 123
Corey, M. S., 112
Cornell, C. P., 63, 80
Costs, in relationships, 22–23
Co-therapy, 4
Counseling, process described, 4–7
Counseling, case examples
    communication issues, 52–56
    ethical issues, 120–123
    gender role issues, 86–88
    love issues, 32–36
    relationship satisfaction, 69–72
    remarried families, 107–109
Couple counseling. *See also* Close
        relationships
    approaches to, 12–16
    attribution work and, 65
    breakups and, 95–96
    defining the client in, 4
    difficult issues in, 10–12
    ethical issues in, 112–117
    exchange theory and, 22–24
    gender roles and (*see* Gender roles)
    homosexual couples, case examples,
        69–72, 120–123
    improving communication through,
        48–50, 95, 96
    introduction to, 2–4
    Love Attitudes Scale and, 29–30

Couple counseling
    power issues in, 79–81
    remarriage and, 102
    Self-Disclosure Index and, 49–50
    sexual problems and, 37, 40, 42–43
    structuring therapy in, 7–12
    therapeutic relationship in, 4, 6–7
    types of therapy in, 4
Couples
    current definition of, 3–4
    issues in assessing, 10–12
Courtship
    relationship development and, 21–24
    sex during, 38–40
Crises, in couple counseling, 10
Crouter, A. C., 84
Cultural groups
    love attitudes among, 29–30
    relationship satisfaction among, 58
Cupach, W. R., 48, 92, 93
Curran, J. P., 39
Curvilinearity, 60
Custody issues, 99, 100
Cutrona, C. E., 66, 67

Dare, C., 13
Date rape, 43, 81
Dattilio, F. M., 10, 12, 14, 40, 48, 49
Davis, K. E., 24
Deaux, K., 76
DeMaris, A., 51
Demographic information, 7, 9
Dependency, relationship breakup
        and, 97
Derlega, V. J., 5, 19, 44, 45
Diagnosis, initial, in couple counsel-
        ing, 8
Dialectical issues, in close relation-
        ships, 92–93
Dindia, K., 45
Dion, K., 20
Disclosure. *See* Self-disclosure
Divorce. *See also* Breakups; Remar-
        riage
    consequences of, 98–101
    stages of, 96–98
    types of, 96
Domination stage, of conflict, 62
Downey, D. B., 100
Drigotas, S. M., 97, 100
Drug abuse, 11

TO THE OWNER OF THIS BOOK:

We hope that you have found *Close Relationships: What Couple Therapists Can Learn* useful. So that this book can be improved in a future edition, would you take the time to complete this sheet and return it? Thank you.

School and address: ————————————————————

Department: ————————————————————

Instructor's name: ————————————————————

1. What I like most about this book is: ————————————————

————————————————————————————

————————————————————————————

2. What I like least about this book is: ————————————————

————————————————————————————

————————————————————————————

3. My general reaction to this book is: ————————————————

————————————————————————————

4. The name of the course in which I used this book is: ——————————

————————————————————————————

5. Were all of the chapters of the book assigned for you to read? ——————

   If not, which ones weren't? ——————————————————

6. In the space below, or on a separate sheet of paper, please write specific suggestions for improving this book and anything else you'd care to share about your experience in using the book.

————————————————————————————

————————————————————————————

————————————————————————————

————————————————————————————

————————————————————————————

Optional:

Your name: _____   Date: _____

May Brooks/Cole quote you, either in promotion for *Close Relationships: What Couple Therapists Can Learn*, or in future publishing ventures?

Yes: _____   No: _____

Sincerely,

Susan S. Hendrick

FOLD HERE

FOLD HERE

Brooks/Cole is dedicated to publishing quality books for the helping professions. If you would like to learn more about our publications, as well as special offers and discounts, please use this mailer to request our catalogue.

Name: ————————————————————————

Street Address: ————————————————————

City, State, and Zip: ——————————————————

FOLD HERE

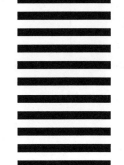

NO POSTAGE
NECESSARY
IF MAILED
IN THE
UNITED STATES

BUSINESS REPLY MAIL
FIRST CLASS   PERMIT NO. 358   PACIFIC GROVE, CA

POSTAGE WILL BE PAID BY ADDRESSEE

ATT: *Human Services Catalogue*

**Brooks/Cole Publishing Company
511 Forest Lodge Road
Pacific Grove, California 93950-9968**

FOLD HERE